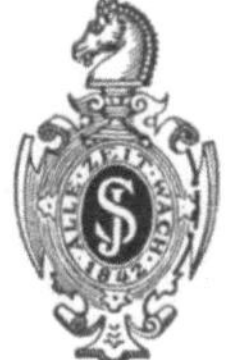

Recent Results in Cancer Research

Fortschritte der Krebsforschung

Progrès dans les recherches sur le cancer

4

Edited by

V. G. Allfrey, New York · M. Allgöwer, Chur · K. H. Bauer, Heidelberg · I. Berenblum, Rehovoth · F. Bergel, London · J. Bernard, Paris · W. Bernhard, Villejuif N. N. Blokhin, Moskva · H. E. Bock, Tübingen · P. Bucalossi, Milano · A. V. Chaklin, Moskva · M. Chorazy, Gliwice · G. J. Cunningham, London · W. Dameshek, Boston M. Dargent, Lyon · G. Della Porta, Milano · P. Denoix, Villejuif · R. Dulbecco, San Diego · H. Eagle, New York · R. Eker, Oslo · P. Grabar, Paris · H. Hamperl, Bonn R. J. C. Harris, London · E. Hecker, Heidelberg · R. Herbeuval, Nancy · J. Higginson, Lyon · W. C. Hueper, Bethesda · H. Isliker, Lausanne · D. A. Karnofsky, New York · J. Kieler, København · G. Klein, Stockholm · H. Koprowski, Philadelphia · L. G. Koss, New York · G. Martz, Zürich · G. Mathé, Paris · O. Mühlbock, Amsterdam · G. T. Pack, New York · V. R. Potter, Madison · A. B. Sabin, Cincinnati · L. Sachs, Rehovoth · E. A. Saxén, Helsinki · W. Szybalski, Madison H. Tagnon, Bruxelles · R. M. Taylor, Toronto · A. Tissières, Genève · E. Uehlinger, Zürich · R. W. Wissler, Chicago · T. Yoshida, Tokyo · L. A. Zilber, Moskva

Editor in chief

P. Rentchnick, Genève

Springer-Verlag Berlin Heidelberg New York 1966

Laser Cancer Research

Leon Goldman

With 42 Figures

Springer-Verlag Berlin Heidelberg New York 1966

*Leon Goldman, M. D., Professor and Chairman Department of Dermatology, College
of Medicine University of Cincinnati and
Director of Medical Laser Laboratories
Children's Hospital Research Foundation and
Medical Center University of Cincinnati, Ohio/USA*

Sponsored by the Swiss League against Cancer

ISBN-13: 978-3-642-87270-9   e-ISBN-13: 978-3-642-87268-6
DOI: 10.1007/978-3-642-87268-6

Introduction

The basic goal of laser research in cancer is to define its value and limitation in cancer research and therapy. This form of radiation, as with other types of radiation, must proceed along the same line and tedious road which x-ray radiation, for example, has followed for so many years. It is hoped that the knowledge of past experiences with x-ray will keep this new flashing darling of the physics laboratory from repeating the same mistakes.

In the field of cancer research, the laser is applied as a type of micro-surgical instrument of great precision for use in investigation in chemistry, cytology, cytogenetics, spectroscopy, and in the treatment of animal experimental cancer. The effect on cancer in animals is produced by absorption of this tremendous high energy and high peak power on both spontaneous and induced tumors. Similar results are produced in cancer of man. Now an effort is made to assess its role in combined programs together with other forms of radiation and of local and systemic cancer chemotherapy agents.

In studies of cancer of man, research in laser is directed to detailed studies of the absorption by different tumors of different types of laser radiation, the immediate and long term effects of the coagulation necrosis induced by the laser and its role as adjunct or synergist to x-ray radiation and cancer chemotherapy agents. Finally, an effort is made now in man to study the effect of the laser on the immunobiology of the cancer.

Experiments on man must be done relatively early in the stage of development of this new complex, sophisticated, and expensive instrumentation, for the optical systems of the tissues of man and also his immunologic mechanisms differ from these in animals.

In brief, it is a tedious painstaking job with continued and necessary co-operation of physicists, engineers, instrument designers, biologists, all working together with the oncologist. For man, the laser must be moved out of the laboratory into the operating room. At present, its true position in the cancer therapy program is not yet known. The greatest attention is being directed to melanoma because of the tremendous energy adsorption capabilities of this heavily pigmented tumor. The next area of interest is in uncommon and common tumors of blood vessels. Here, too, the color factor influences to a significant degree the absorption of the laser. Multiple accessible malignancies are treated also by the laser chiefly to compare the effect here with other modalities of therapy. Finally, as a type of therapy of desperation, lasers are used in the treatment of metastatic lesions.

This then, is the brief introduction to the study of the current status of laser cancer research. Intense, difficult and cooperative research of the next few years will determine the role of the laser, an „optical knife", as an investigative or therapeutic instrument.

Table of Contents

Chapter 1

Laser Instrumentation

For many biologists and physicists, laser technology opens up an entirely new, strange and even wonderful field. It is well to review the basic concepts of radiation physics before considering the actual laser instrumentation.

Some of the definitions to recall are such simple terms as energy, energy density, power and coherency. Energy is the ability to do work and is expressed as joules. Energy density is the energy concentration per unit area to be expressed as joules per square centimeter. Power is the work done per unit of time and is expressed as (watts per second). High energy density and high power characterize laser radiation.

Conventional sources of light are incoherent. Laser light is coherent. That is, it has spatial and temporal simultaneity groups of light waves.

The laser beam is monochromatic, coherent and has direction, since the light can be focused by any lens system and finally it has tremendous high energy and high power. The duration of the laser beam impact may vary from milliseconds to billionths of a second, from 10^{-3} to 10^{-9} seconds.

The following tables are of interest:

One joule equals 9.485×10^{-4} B.T.U.
One joule equals 10^7 ergs
One joule equals 2.39×10^{-3} gram calories
One joule equals 6.738 foot pounds
One gram calorie equals 4.185 joules
One B.T.U. equals 1045 joules
One electron volt (e.d.) equals 1.602×10^{-2} ergs

Wave length conversion

One Å equals 10^{-10} meters
One Å equals 3.937×10^{-9} inches
One Å equals 10^{-4} microns
One Å equals 10^{-1} millimicrons
One micron equals 39.37 microinches
One mil (0.001 inch) equals 25.4 microns

The principal of the laser then is essentially a system which optically pumps a mass and excites the atoms to a higher energy and as the energy drops there is stimulated emission of radiation. That word LASER is an acronym and is obtained from Light Amplification by Stimulated Emission of Radiation. At present, 300 laser wave lengths in 23 elements are available for the continuous wave gas lasers.

Various types of lasers which are of interest, primarily for the biomedical aspects
are:

1. the solid crystal laser—ruby and neodymium
2. the gas laser—argon, carbon dioxide, helium-neon,
3. the junction diode.

As yet, the liquid lasers, chelate type or free rare earth ions in inorganic solvents,
have not been used in biomedical research. A type of solid laser, a synthetic ruby rod,
is pumped by light from the xenon flash tubes arranged in a highly reflective cavity
to direct the output on to the rod. This absorbed energy is transformed into monchro-
matic, coherent, high intensity laser light. The ruby crystal is a carrier of aluminum
oxide with chromium atoms added forming the lattice work. One end of the rod
forms a 100% reflector, the other end of the optical cavity is partially transparent.
The ruby laser in its light of the wave length is 6943 Å. The efficiency of this system
is very low. To increase efficiency of output, cooling systems are used such as liquid
nitrogen, water and circulating refrigerants. For repeatable outputs, the temperature
of the rod should be as constant as possible.

The neodymium laser, the other important type of solid laser for high energy
biomedical research is a glass which is doped with neodymium. This emits light in
wave lengths of 10,600 Å. The neodymium laser, since it is made of glass, is much
easier to make in large sizes than the ruby laser and it has an efficiency which is
higher than the ruby laser. For example, large size neodymium glass approximately
$3/4'' \times 30''$ long has a 3% efficiency rating. The ruby, in much smaller sizes has an
efficiency rating of between one and two per cent.

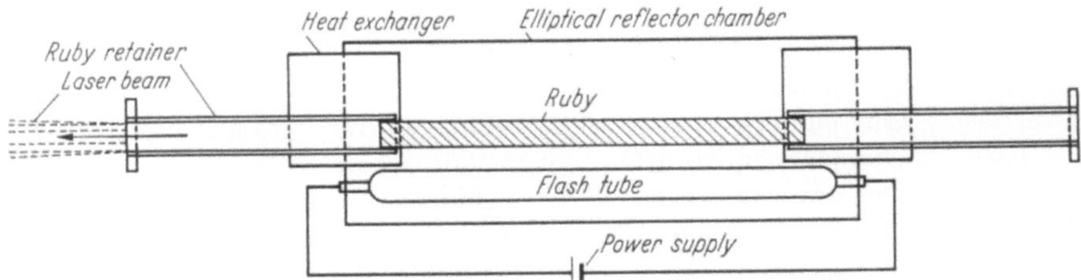

Fig. 1. Basic design of pulsed ruby laser

Some of the problems that relate to the use of the laser biomedical applications
include flexibility of the instruments, to be able to be used off the optical bench and
the fact that for laser cancer work, high energy lasers must be used, at least 50 joules
of exit energy. The linear flash lamps which we use are xenon and supply the power
to pump the solid crystals. As the energy requirement increases, the flash lamps break
much easier and become weaker. Also, great sources of electrical energy supplies the
currents that are needed. These basic features of equipment, the capacitor blanks to
supply electrical energy, the flash lights, the laser rods with their cavities all make for
very expensive, sophisticated equipment. To help in cancer research, the laser industry
must develop better rods, more reliable flash tubes, and optical instrumentation to
transmit or reflect laser beams.

There is another type of laser radiation which is of considerable interest for biomedical applications. This is the Q-switching or Q-spoiling. In the regular emission,

the duration of the laser pulse is relatively long in milliseconds. However, the light can be stored temporarily in the optical cavity and then allowed suddenly to break out as a giant pulse wave. In this technique, the transmission mirror of the laser rod is replaced by a rotating fused quartz prism which contributes reflectivity to the optical cavity. Or a Kerr cell shutter may be used. Also used is a cell containing a bleachable dye which contributes to saturation of the light in the cavity. This bleachable dye may include various dyes such as thallium cyanide and nitrobenzine, Eastman's dye 9740 UPI or other types. The cell with dye and the rotating prism may be combined together.

In the Q-switching technique, the peak power outputs are measured in megawatts and may reach even into gigawatts. Under these tremendous impacts of power highly selective rods are needed to maintain the instrument. The biomedical studies of Q-

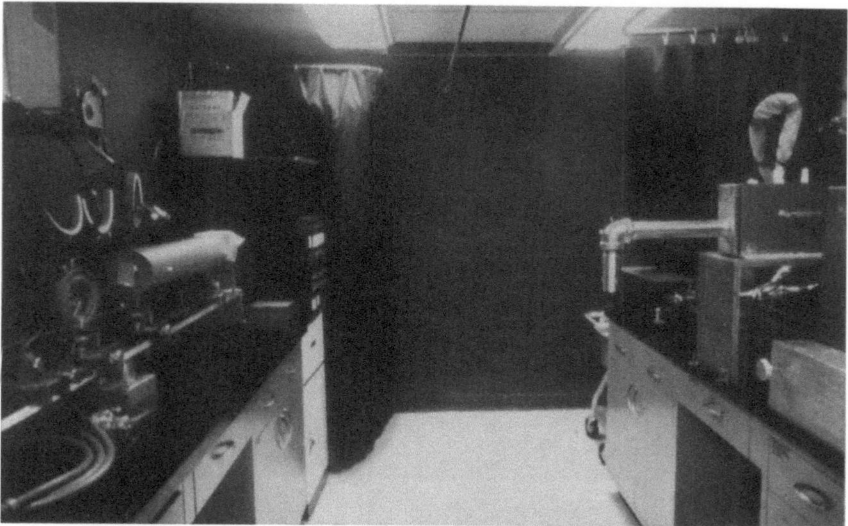

Fig. 2. Laser Laboratory, Children's Hospital Research Foundation, Cincinnati, Ohio, U.S.A., showing air cooled neodymium laser (Eastman) exit energy 200 joules and liquid nitrogen cooled ruby laser (Maser Optics Inc.) 80 joules exit energy with gold mirror attachment (Western Electric) to reflect laser beam

switching are really just beginning to be studied. Powers of 10 megawatts peak power output have temporarily bleached tatoos on the skin. One-hundred megawatts peak power outputs have caused slight punctures of the skin. A laser physicist is said to have had an accidental impact of 500 megawatts peak power output on the dorsum of his hand with only mild atrophy and temporary hair loss resulting.

One of the features of the impact of the laser on living tissue is the development of a plume or plasma cloud on the target area. The appearance of that means that there has been absorption of laser energy by the target area. The components of this will be discussed in the mechanism of the laser action on the skin.

The gas laser uses gas for lasing. This produces a constant wave, C.W., unlike the pulsed emission of the ruby and neodymium lasers. Almost any type of gas can be used. For example, helium-neon gas combination produces 6328 Å. Until recently, the output of gas lasers was weak and had very little biomedical aspects, except for

1*

certain work in tissue cultures. However, recently, especially with the argon gas laser and the carbon dioxide, nitrogen molecular laser, higher power outputs have been produced. Cancer studies with the use of the high output C.W. lasers are just beginning. The argon laser 4880 Å—5145 Å does have some selective effect on pigment and blood vessels. The carbon dioxide laser 106,000 Å, has chiefly thermal effect but some effect against hemorrhage with high power outputs of 50 watts or more. The advantages of the gas laser is that unlike the solid state laser the laser beams are not pulsed, but they are constant on the target. Although laser technology is attempting to increase the frequency of laser impacts by the use of so-called repetitive lasers, impacts in terms of seconds or fractions of a second, the advantage of the gas lasers is that there is a continuous laser impact directed to the tumor. The light beam here functions as an optical knife.

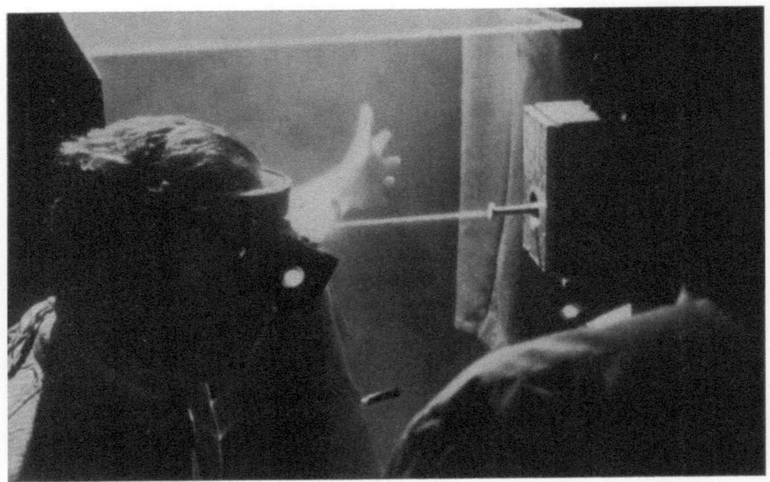

Fig. 3. Impact of pulsed ruby laser vaporizing mark of India ink on forearm and producing no effect on the skin. Beam made visible by transmission through a cloud of incense. Exit energy 15 joules

The junction diodes have been used very little in biomedical work at the present time because of the low output and the need to operate at liquid hydrogen or at helium temperatures. However, this type because of its simplicity, efficiency and small size does have tremendous possibilities if they can be developed for use at room temperatures and for high outputs. In this type of laser, an electric current instead of light across the p-n junction of a semi-conductor such as gallium a arsenide, pumps materials in the semi-conductor to emit photons. These photons may come out as coherent light. This is an example then, of the "transference" of electrons into protons. Instead of unreliable light sources as with the solid state lasers, electric currents are used.

One of the many difficulties of laser instrumentation for biomedical applications is the difficulty of measurement of laser output. Measurement should be done in the same fashion that standardized measurements are done for the calibration of x-ray radiation. If laser measurements cannot be standardized, then it is difficult to compare or analyze the results of laser therapy of cancer.

In brief, energy of laser radiation can be measured by the following methods:

1. thermal
2. mechanical
3. photoelectric.

These measurements can be made in brief by a beam splitter taking off a known portion of the laser beam and submitting it to measuring instrumentation. Thermal measurements are done by absorption in a calorimeter, usually copper cone, "rat nest" type or liquid cell type. This is not too effective for very high energy measurement or for Q-switching.

Mechanical measurements are made with impact pressure usually from the impact on the mirror with the wire attachment developing torque and the subsequent measurement of torsion.

Photoelectric instruments measure the light produced by the laser. High energy and high power outputs, which may destroy or damage the light cell, brief duration of the pulses, unstandardized instrumentation are but some of the factors involved. Too few outside of the field of laser technology seem to appreciate the great need for instrumentation research in this area of laser output measurements.

In listing the dosage received, it is well to describe it as

1. the laser which is used
2. the output, with its wave lengths
3. the lens system used
4. the target area which is used
5. the energy density
6. the characteristics of the pulse duration and whether the pulse goes up slow or gradually, whether it has single or multiple spikes
7. the light transmission system.

These later features may be measured and portrayed by the oscilloscope.

One other feature of laser technology of interest in biomedical work is the production of second harmonics. In this instance, the laser wave length is cut in half and even thirds or fourths by passage through various types of crystal material such as potassium dihydrogen phosphate and lithium niobate or even amino acids. Second harmonics may produce some biomedical aspects from the ruby laser or from the neodymium. For example, second harmonic radiation from the ruby may produce ultraviolet laser radiation. The biological effects of second harmonics have been used only in initial studies, such as in cytology and cytogenetics and in impacts of DNA and of skin, both normal and pathologic.

To attempt to make the laser more flexible, various techniques are used to transmit the laser beam from the laser head. These include lenses, prisms, mirrors especially gold and silver mirrors, gaseous thermal gradients, dielectric tubes, quartz rods and tubes and even clear plastics.

The laser attached to a microscope or reflected from an external source through a microscope is an excellent and efficient instrument to study effects of the laser in cytology and cytogenetics. The laser beam is transmitted through the optics of the microscope on to the cellular material. BESSIS and also MALT, who have done so much work in this field, have been able to focus the beam down to one micron. Here, energy densities between 10^{-5} to 10^{-1} joules/micron^2 (10^3—10^7 joules/cm^2) are sufficient (STORB). This makes for a highly selective microsurgical instrument which can be used on individual portions of the cell such as the nucleus or even in mito-

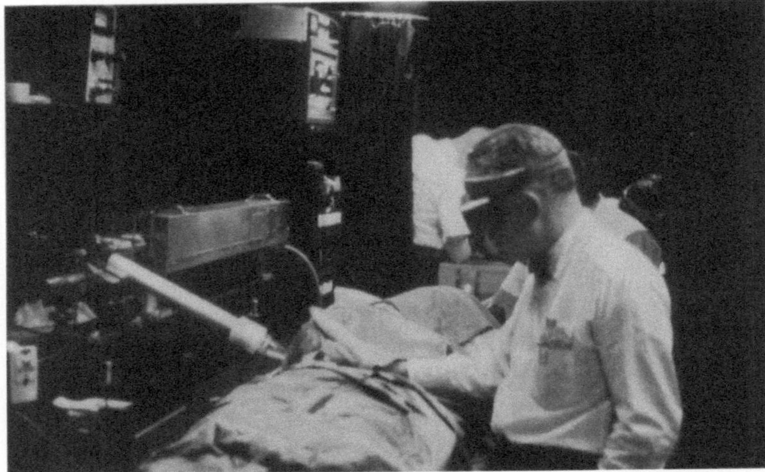

Fig. 4. Picture of experimental laboratory model Eastman neodymium laser exit energy 1160 joules with quartz prism attachment to direct laser beam on to metastatic melanoma of the lower abdominal wall

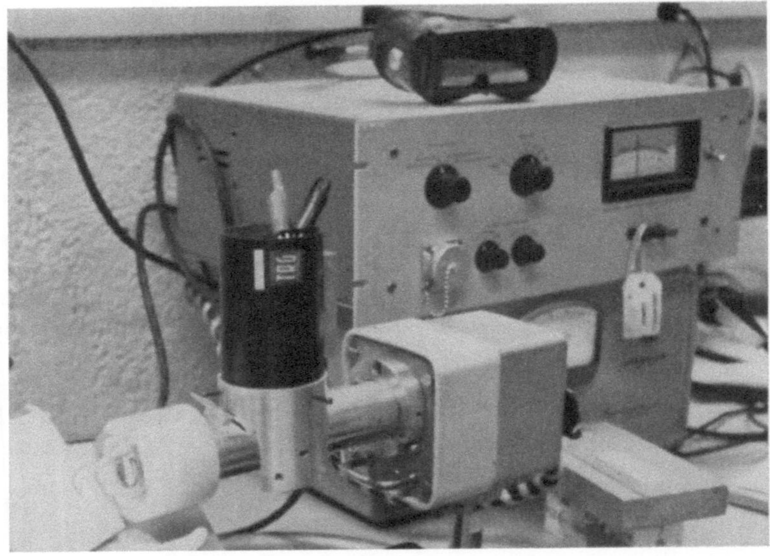

Fig. 5. Measurement of output of low energy of pulsed ruby laser (Maser Optics, Inc.) with beam splitter and copper cone T.R.G. Calorimeter

chondria. ROUNDS and his associates have shown the great value of the laser microscope in cancer research.

Another instrument of great importance is the laser microprobe. This instrument is in brief a laser, modified Q-switching type, attached to a microscope. The material is put in the microscope stage. The plume developed in the laser impact completes the arc between two carbon electrodes, and this is then passed through the lens system to the spectroscope. This technique developed by BRECH and ROSAN enables one to do

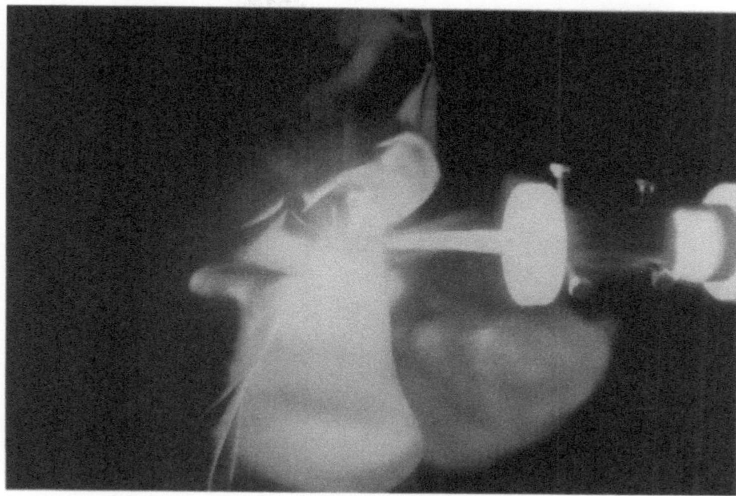

Fig. 6. Impact of ruby laser transmitted through curved quartz rod producing 650 joules/cm² of energy density for treatment of superficial malignancy of back. Black and white copy of Infrared Ektachrome (Eastman) picture of actual impact showing plume, coloring of quartz rod and intense reflectance from target area

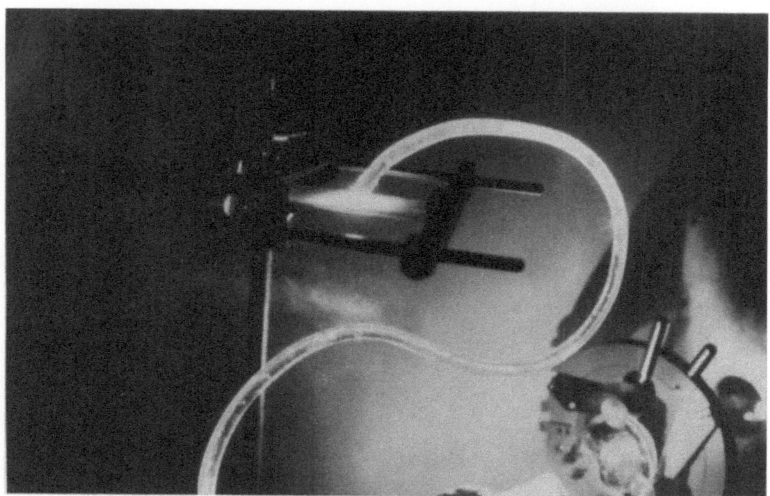

Fig. 7. Showing passage of low energy ruby laser through curved clear epoxy rods with destruction of red cells in fresh blood smear in contact with exit end

direct spectroscopy of small selected areas of living tissue. In the field of cancer research, the laser microprobe permits spectroscopic analysis of selected areas of living cancer tissue, without the complete destruction of the sample. A continued development of this apparatus as regards quantitation will provide a valuable instrument for cancer research.

In all phases of laser technology the biologist and the physician must work with the engineer and the physicist. Laser instrumentation has not reached the desired state of maturity yet, and it is not the least bit, an assembly-lone product. Its use must be monitored often by the physicist and by the engineer. Progress in the development of laser techniques is very necessary for laser surgery. An efficient laser surgery operating room will be made possible only by such combined co-operative efforts. This need for co-operative research will continue for some time in the biomedical applications of the laser.

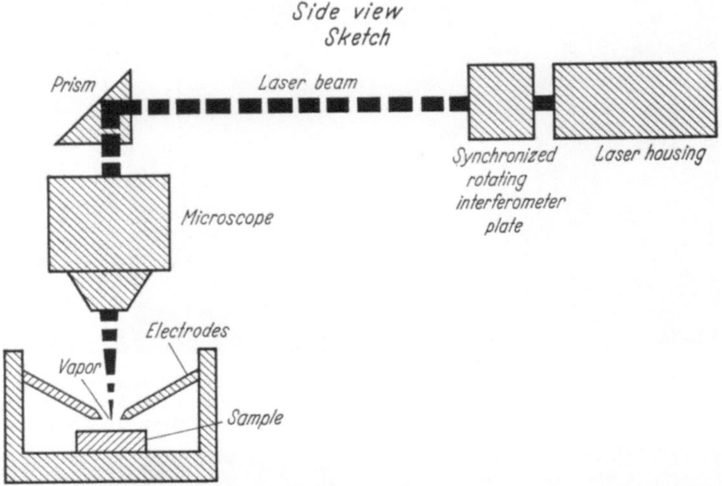

Fig. 8. Laser microprobe with Q-switched laser attachment for laser spectroscopy of living tissue (FREDERICK BRECH)

High energy laser systems are of necessity complicated and expensive and for cancer research will be limited at present to large medical centers. Low energy lasers for basic research and lasers attached to microscopes can be used quite properly and often in the well equipped cancer research laboratory.

The future of laser research depends upon the continued adaption of new advances in modifications of laser technology. Advances in the immunobiology of cancer, the continued basic research in cancer all will have to be applied to the controlled clinical observations of cancer patients treated by the laser. The development of international committees for the study of laser radiation, especially laser radiation of cancer, will make for the more rapid advances and furnish data for critical analysis of the distinct values and the very distinct limitations of this form of radiation in the field of cancer research.

Chapter 2
Laser Protection

Laser radiation is a form of electromagnetic radiation and so there must be both area and personal protection. One does not wish to repeat the tragic story of the early days of x-ray radiation in its application to medicine. High energy laser radiation is required in cancer research especially in man. This high energy and high peak power requirement increases the problem of protection.

The basic needs of protection is especially the eye. Then follows the protection of the exposed tissues and then the inhalation hazards through aerosol particles of the plume, charged particles (?), the nitrogen oxides, from the nitrogen coolants when they are used. Because the high power electrical requirements are needed, there is always the hazard of electrical burns and shock.

Fig. 9. Laser sign to be used in all areas where laser radiation is given (modified after DE MENT)

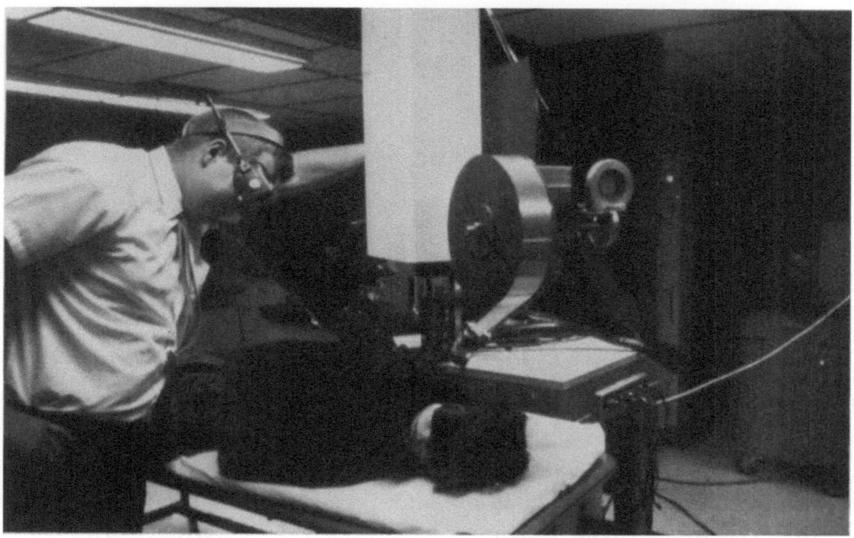

Fig. 10. Protective glasses worn by personnel and patient during the charging of the laser for laser treatment of angioma of face

The first requirement for clinical laser research is the development and construction of the laser laboratory. This means adequate planning area control of laser radiation. In essence, this is the construction of a special biomedical laser laboratory, not merely the adaptation of a convenient corner or, more often, an inconvenient corner of a laboratory.

For lasers attached to microscopes, area control is centered about the microscope. Equipment must be devised to protect the operator from the laser beam which is reflected through the ocular system of the microscope or reflected from an external source into the microscope. Protection from the beam may be secured by the imposition of a metal plate on the microscope when the laser is being charged. The complete enclosure of the laser attachment to the microscope also adds additional protection for the operator. Least desirable is the need to have the operator to turn the head away when firing of the laser.

The same requirements hold for the laser microprobe for laser spectroscopy. In the past it was somewhat the custom to check the laser microprobe impact with the operator's own finger. This should not be done, since control studies may be done by the direct impact of black film or a metal sheet.

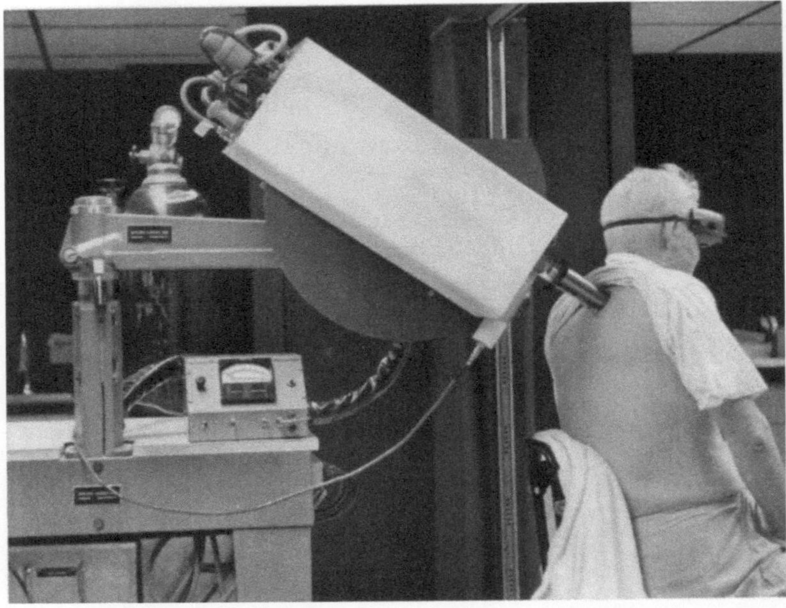

Fig. 11. Special laser treatment room painted with dull black surfaces, warning lights and door locks in Laser Laboratory, Children's Hospital Research Foundation, Cincinnati, Ohio, U.S.A. Water cooled high energy ruby laser (Applied Lasers Inc.) with flexible mount and enclosed lens systems. Laser treatment for epithelioma of upper back. Protective glasses worn by patient

The design of the laser treatment room especially for high energy laser equipment is the construction of a specific area in which the operator and the patient are both protected. The room should be appropriately marked, preferrably with the laser danger sign on the door. With the charging of the high energy laser system no one else should be allowed in the room besides the attendants needed in the actual laser treatment. Often laser treatment rooms are painted black with diffuse types of coating in an attempt to cut down the reflectivity of the laser beam. The isolation of the laser area, so that no other work besides the actual laser treatment goes on in that area, is important. In this manner, personnel will not wander carelessly into an area in which the laser is firing.

If possible, the control panel and the cable should not be in the same room so that the operator of the laser equipment is not subject to repeated exposures. The patient and all personnel in the laser treatment area should be provided with effective protective glasses. These will be discussed in detail later. The actual treatment or target area should be protected so that there is no undue exposure other than the actual treatment area.

The black drapes absorb a significant amount although BUCKLEY claims they may not be as effective for the high energy neodymium radiation. Green drapes may be used for neodymium treatments. Carboard is an effective protectant of the area which it is desired not to radiate. The specific requirements for protection form undesired transmission escape, reflectance, etc., with the use of quartz rods, quartz glass tubes, prisms and gold mirrors will be described for the specific experiments.

The eye is the most significant organ to be considered in laser radiation. Eye damage from radiation has been known according to HAM ever since the time of GALEN in 200 BC. GALILEO is said to have injured his eye through continued observation with his famous telescope. The eye damages from the atomic blasts are well known. Because the pigment of the eye and the lens of the eye, the laser radiation can be focused in the eye and even low energy densities may produce severe damage. Such accidents have occurred in the laser laboratories. An accident to a laser physicist has been reported by RATHKEY. Carelessness, premature discharge of unreliable flash tubes, reflection from the spectral surfaces are some of the factors influencing eye damage. Even with continuous wave lasers with weak outputs should there by any undue exposure of the eye. Low energy laser impacts on the eye may be similar to the severage damage from intense white lights such as xenon light. Recently high output argon and carbon dioxide lasers have been used in cancer research. Eye protection is difficult here since the usual laser protec-

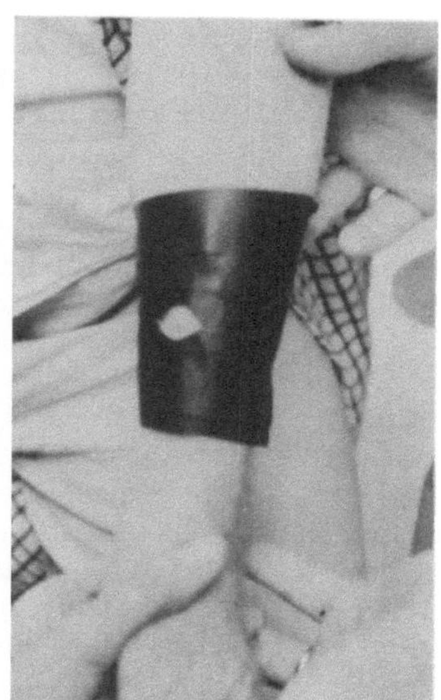

Fig. 12 Showing black paper protecting forearm for laser treatment of superficial squamous carcinoma

tive glasses are not effective and prolonged use of the laser is made. At present, we have used an amber colored plastic plate to protect our eyes in cancer surgery with an experimental model CW argon laser, 4 watt output, on loan from Bell Telephone Laboratories. For high output carbon dioxide lasers, any glass can protect.

Again it is emphasized that the eyes must be protected at all times. This means the development of an effective comfortable type of laser protective glasses. In brief, the glasses used in biomedical laser resarch are a type of soft welder's frame glasses with complete close fitting so that there is no possibility of exposure from the sides or from the back. In general, the first coverage for protection is a shield of clear glass, sometimes with magnification although magnification increases the desire to get closer to the target area to define the detailed features of the target mass. On top of this first layer of glass is the filter glass, of appropriate thickness, and something for the appropriate laser radiation. Schott BG glass No. 18 is used for protection against ruby and neodymium laser. It is important to emphasize that there is no universal single protective filter. Recently in our laboratory RITTER has developed a protective glass containing an occlusive shutter. Only after this is closed can the laser fire. This protective eye shield can not be used with CW lasers. For ruby and for neodymium the shot BG 18 glass is effective. This is not effective for ultraviolet lasers, where a blue filter must be interposed. Little is known about eye protection for the powerful argon laser. In high energy laser work the glasses should be worn during the charging of the apparatus since premature flashing may produce severe eye damage. In case of any accident, an ophthalmologist should be consulted immediately. Eyes should not be rubbed after an accidental exposure because rubbing of the burned cornea may induce severe reaction.

Personnel in the laser laboratory, depending upon the degree of exposure, should have eye examination by the ophthalmologist in the laser group at least every six months. The examination should include a detailed exam, fundus picture and slit lamp.

Little is known about the effect of chronic exposure to the eye. This is important for laser personnel who may be exposed to reflection of the laser beam for prolonged periods of time. A constant reappraisal of protection program in a laser laboratory should be done at intervals.

The patient to be treated should also be protected with the same type of glasses, and should be given instruction of the need for closing the eyes, as well as the use of glasses. For impacts about the face, other additional coverings of the eye may be used underneath the laser glasses, black cloth for ruby impacts, green cloth for neodymium impacts. Continued research is being done on significant features of transillumination, and tissues about the eye, to determine whether any significant damage to the eye may occur in the actual transillumination of tissues.

There is no substitue for the use of protective glasses. Merely closing the eye, leaves only the dubious filtration of the very thin and transparent eyelid. Turning the head away does not insure against the reflected beams. The use of higher and higher energy densities increases the need for continued concern about the eye protection.

The next significant feature is the plume. The plume arises from the impact of the laser on the target. This plume of high temperatures is composed of free radicals (?), charged particles (?), and aerosol fragments (?). Aerosol particles may be scattered to a significant degree about the area of impact depending upon the energy density. These aerosol particles may be of various bits of the charred or changed tissue. Tumor fragments are still viable. Production of ionization, this especially with Q-switching, is still under investigation. The enclosure of the laser system, the continued research and the development of plume traps may reduce the hazards by the plume.

In small laboratory spaces where significant amounts of nitrogen coolants may be employed, the reduction of oxygen concentration in the air may be a significant. This can be checked with determination of oxygen concentration in the air. At present nitrogen is not used very much.

The problem of the ionization of air, especially from high peak power Q-switching, is still unsettled. Continued studies are being done on this feature. Because of this possibility, the examination of personnel as regards complete blood counts in addition to eye examination will serve as a control in this particular feature.

Especially with experimental high energy laser laboratory models with high power electrical current, there is a constant hazard of electric burn and shock. The problem of electric sparking should also be considered in the use of the laser in the operating rooms where explosive gases may be used anywhere in the operating areas.

Added to the usual complex problem of laser protection is the prevention program for laser surgery in the sterile atmosphere of the hospital operating unit. Here the laser head must be kept clean, the lens system covered by moving protective glass or tape as HARDWAY has suggested to avoid splattering from the plume. This will avoid bacterial contamination of the laser wound. Special quartz rods will localize the laser beam to target areas and reduce the hazards somewhat. Protective screens about the operating table should be used. The demonstration laser surgical operating room at the National Cancer Institute under Ketchum will serve as a model for the development of similar units over the country.

Chapter 3
The Laser Reaction in Tissue

The development of the laser brought to the biologist and to the cancer researcher a form of radiation from the visible end of the spectrum. For the first time, there were available light waves which produced tremendous power and energy densities. The laser reaction in tissue produces a multi-faceted response. A large part of this reaction is thermal, some of it is physical, and some is what may be called loosely, electromagnetic.

The thermal reaction is an important phase of the response to the laser. The characteristic picture of the laser impact is a brilliant flash with vaporization of tissue. Photography shows the bright light of the impact together with a bright cloud called the plume. The surface of the impact is charred with the degree of destruction depending upon the energy density. According to BRECH, the plume has a high temperature, an abundance of excited atoms, a few ions, a few electrons and has considerable pressure. Also, in addition, we have observed aerosol particles of various sizes and shapes depending upon the area which is impacted. This plume is of great significance when it develops in a closed cavity such as the eye, cranial mouth or pleural or abdominal cavities of the body. The effect on the target area is that of a charring, which on superficial inspection is simply that of the heat type of reaction. The brief duration of the laser impact in terms of milliseconds down to nanoseconds is often responsible for the sharply demarcated quality of the local laser response in tissue. Conduction and convection spread this thermal reaction.

Ultra-sonic and recoil pressure waves are induced in tissue by the impact. These may be shown by high-speed photography of the target area. Occasionally, these pressure waves may be seen in the impact of the laser on agar blocks colored with ink when the impact is observed under the microscope. Holography and micro-holography are being used to study these stresses in tissue.

With various types of transducers, sonic, ultra-sonic, and even hyper-sonic waves may be detected in tissue. With thermocouple arrangements and the effective materials covering the transducers, KLINE and FINE have established that it is the pressure which is producing the sonic reactions not the radiation itself. So, added to the thermal effect in tissue is the effect on the cells of pressure and sonic vibration.

Especially with the production of high energy and high peak power outputs, various types of reactions loosely described as electromagnetic may develop in tissues.

Free radical formation can be detected by electron spin resonance spectrometry. It is supposed that these develop after considerable disturbance of the molecule. Whether other types of heavy particles are developed in addition to the free radical formation is not certain as yet, but apparently some investigators have described the heavy particle formation after laser impact. In brief however, the thermal changes are the most important.

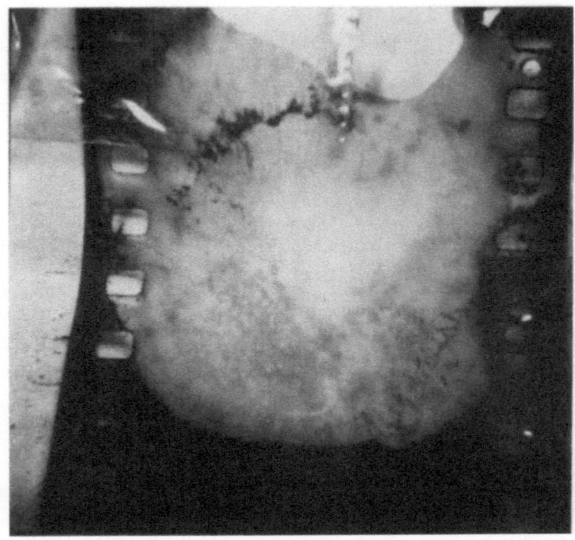

a

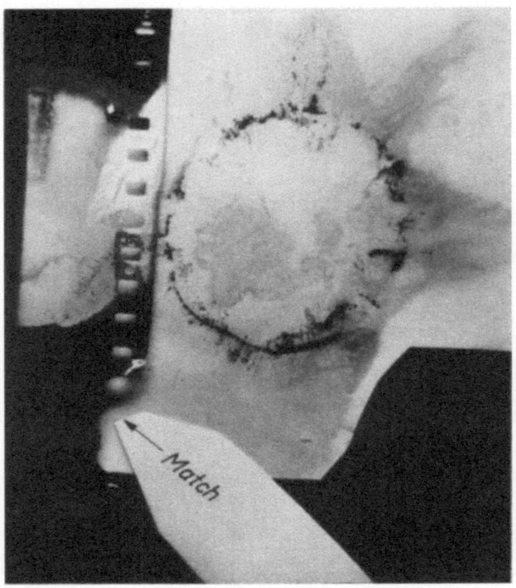

b

Fig. 13 a. Showing removal of silver from film sheet without burning of film. 600 joules exit energy pulsed ruby laser. b. Deposit of silver was deposited on white paper in back of film. Match burn of film strip visible in lower portion

Enzyme changes may be produced as a result of laser impact even though experiments with in vitro exposure of colorless enzyme solution to laser impacts have shown no significant changes. Heat induced in tissue may, however, affect enzyme systems. From the amino acids present in tissue, second harmonics may develop. This then is another form of radiation induced by the laser impact. When second harmonics are in the ultraviolet band there may be significant effect on DNA.

Evidently then, the laser reaction in tissue is a complex series of events both not only at the time of the initial impact, but also as the reaction progresses. The high water content of fluid, some 70% in skin and some 75% in muscle, 70% in liver, and 80—90% in the brain, for example, limits the thermal reaction to the localized area of impact because of the short duration of this impact. Other reactions, however, may develop and progress from the target area. Thus the tissue reactions continue from the area calculated for the target. This has been noted especially in pigmented lesions such as melanomas. Other mechanisms under recent study are the two photon absorption in a single event, inverse Bremsstrahlung and non-linear scattering phenomena.

The progressive necrosis after laser impact is of considerable interest. In addition to the physical and the electromagnetic changes which may be responsible for the extension of the laser reaction, the possibility of spreading thrombosis through the impact of the laser is real. This develops from damage to the blood cells in the tumor area.

The late response to the laser is not known as yet. In our studies of normal and pathologic tissue impacted by the laser, the period of observation is only some three years. The picture is that of a non-specific fibrosis. There is no resemblance to post radiation changes in the blood vessels or in collagen.

The differences between the tissue reactions from the various types of lasers in relation to the cancer research is not completely known at present. The neodymium laser may have less surface impact compared to the ruby laser of the same energy density but there may be significantly more penetration of the neodymium laser. This we have shown with melanomas. The argon and the carbon dioxide lasers may produce significant thermal reactions in tissue. The depth of penetration studies with these continuous wave lasers is as yet unknown.

Q-switching techniques with tremendous peak power outputs may have more significant pressure and expecially electromagnetic reactions. This is not established fully as yet. Efforts to prove the production of ionization of tissue other than free radical formation, such as by film badge techniques, scintillation counter and actual cloud chamber analysis have shown nothing definite in our laboratories as yet, for Q-switching at least up to 125 megawatts of peak power output. Whether these negative findings will hold for outputs of gigawatts and with counters of greater sensitivity and more rapid response is not known yet. All these factors are important to cancer research because it is in high energy and high peak field that the cancer therapy programs in man will be directed.

There is another factor which must be considered in the analysis of the laser reaction. The effect of the penetration of the laser beam in relationship to adjacent and significant structures. For lesions over blood vessels, nerves, bony prominences, joint surfaces, pleural cavity, brain and the like, the question of penetration of the laser impact must be considered. Now, the laser beam can be focused by lens systems to depths in tissue. These factors should be considered in the planning of the details of laser impact. The laser reaction as indicated, depends upon not only the exit energy or power which is delivered to the target area and density but also upon the characteristics of the target area. The characteristics of the target area are essentially those of a biological-optical system — color increasing the absorption of the laser beam, the heterogeneity of the system, and influencing dispersion and reflection. If some areas of the tumor, then, have different optical qualities, there will be different effects of the laser. As the beam penetrates deeper and deeper into tissue, the energy is attenuated and these factors must be also considered in evaluation of the tissue depth of the laser response.

It has not been established whether laser reaction in tissue is more susceptible to secondary infection as yet, but the lesions should be treated as is the therapy for a deep and persistent coagulation necrosis.

Another field of significance in the analysis of the laser reaction is the immuno-biological response of the laser necrosis. It is not know as yet whether there are any specific features to this at all. Does the laser impact on tissue produce a different type of antibody than an ordinary burn? This is under study at the present time. In certain features of cancer research the partial electrosurgery of cancer of the rectum has been said to produce some type of therapy which is used as a comparative treatment to laser therapy in a rough attempt as a control. No immune response is shown as yet with the laser reaction, although Klein and Fine have shown difficulty of reinoculation with melanoma in some animals after laser necrosis of the melanoma.

The delayed response to the laser reaction characteristic in some of the cancers which we have treated at the present time, such as basal cell epitheliomas, can be explained upon local tissue response, rather than in the development of immune reaction. The effects on gamma globulin of laser radiation may have some significance also in the study of the immune response. The inflammatory infiltrate about the laser reaction is non-specific in type, offering no proof as yet of the development of any immune reaction. In brief, then, there is a coagulation necrosis induced by the laser. The immediate picture is fairly well established. The late response is not completely known as yet.

The recent development of laser instrumentation of higher and higher energy and power outputs may change this picture. Laser then, is still an investigative tool in basic cancer research and in clinical investigative studies. Incomplete knowledge of the laser reaction in tissues of both man and animals establishes the need for clinical observation in all phases of the laser therapy. This includes also the continued follow-up of the patient and the need for repeated biopsy studies, and critical analyses of other therapeutic techniques.

Chapter 4

Color Qualities of Tissues in Relation to Laser Radiation

With the lasers now available, color is an important property for the absorption of the incident laser beam. Absorption means destruction of tissue by the laser. This does occur to some extent even in so-called transparent tissues which may show some reaction to the absorptive laser beam. The mechanism here is thought to be two-photon absorption. The incident beam of the laser striking tissue may be reflected, absorbed or transmitted. The darker the tissue, the more absorption and the less reflection and transmission. Reflection of the laser beam may produce reactions on both patient and personnel about the impact. Transmission may occur as the same frequency or if second or other harmonics are produced in tissue, as different frequencies. In addition, as indicated previously, absorption may produce not

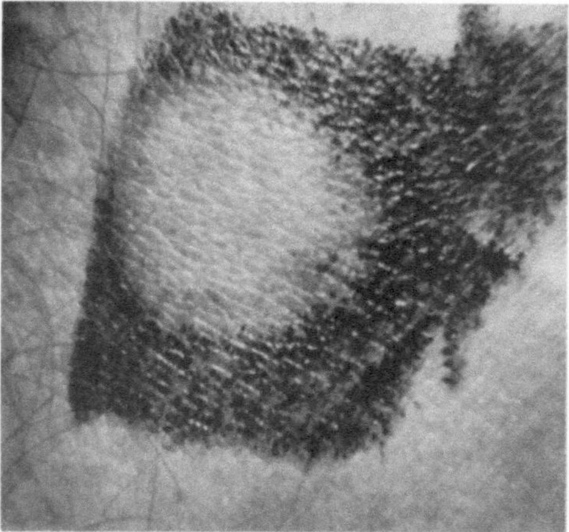

Fig. 14. Removal of India ink from surface of forearm of a Caucasian by unfocussed beam of pulsed ruby laser exit energy 15 joules without any burning or discomfort to the skin

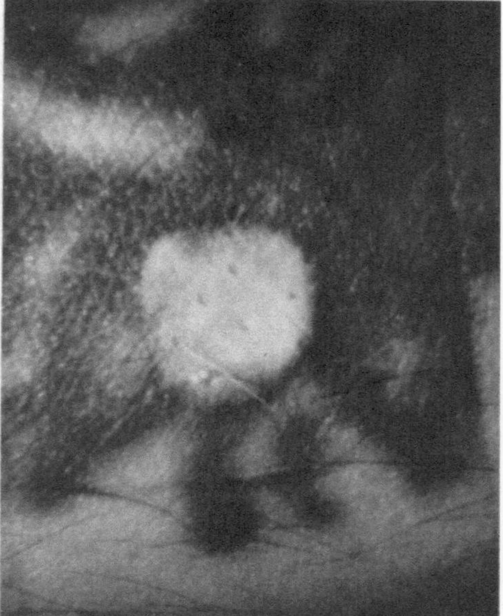

Fig. 15. Transient white blanching in tattoo. Q-switched ruby laser peak power output 20 megawatts

only a thermal reaction but may give rise to such mechanical phenomena as the pressure waves, sonic waves and finally what is vagualy calles "electromagnetic changes".

The more intense and darker the color then, the greater the absorption. This can be shown in tissue culture techniques and in clinical investigative studies. The extent of coagulation necrosis depends on energy densities and power densities on the surface and in depths of tissue. In general, the more pigmented the mass is the more intense will be the coagulation necrosis in the more superficial parts of the mass. If a

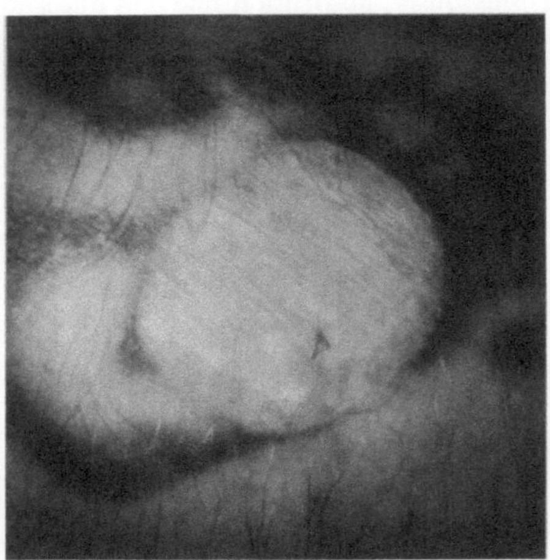

laser beam is focused at depths in the tissue, the intensity of coagulation necrosis will not be as marked in the more superficial portions as it would be deeper in tissue if the same optical qualities of the tissue mass are found in the deeper areas.

Color functions then as a black body absorber of the photons. If tissue does not have pigment, pigment may be given to it artifically by dyes. That is why chemical studies of the effect of lasers on dyes are important.

In man, the melanin and the hemoglobin are effective absorbers of laser radiation. Melanin is changed and vaporizes. As yet, there has been no electromicroscopic or chemical studies of the melanin change. Melanin is the more effective absorber of laser radiation in man. The curious paradox about hemo-

Fig. 16. Scar of tattoo following impact of unfocussed beam of neodymium laser 320 joules exit energy one year previously. Biopsy of scar showed non-specific fibrosis with fragments of tattoo pigments

globin is that although it absorbs laser radiation in itself, there is very little change. This has been shown by the studies of KLINE and FINE and by FORRISTAL in our laboratory. Red cells are sensitive to laser impact in energy densities of the order

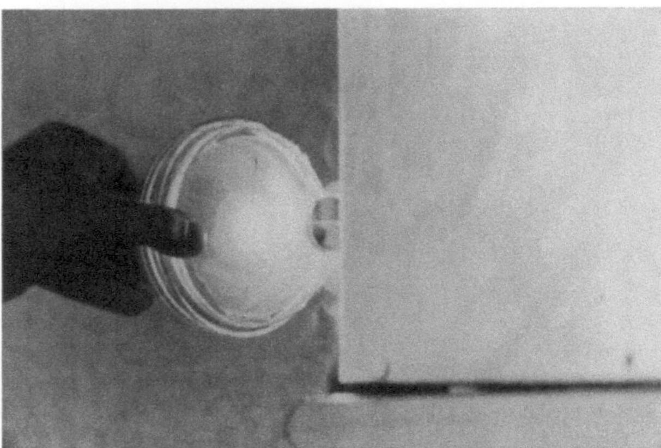

Fig. 17. Chromogenic mycobacterium on agar plate used to study influence of color on absorption of laser

0.1—2 joules per square centimeter. Total destruction and vacuolization in varying degrees are produced in the red cells. In laser microscope, BESSIS has shown the dynamic pictures of the phagocytosis and hemorrhage. The absorption of the laser by the blood velles is one of the reasons why fresh tissue must be used to study the effects of lasers.

From the impacts of the Caucasian skin of man, the pulsed ruby laser produces the more significant changes in the basal cell layer (melanocytes) and in the superficial blood vessels. This so-called selective absorption is found with the low energy densities of wide range 100—200 joules per square centimeter. High energy densities produce diffuse charring of the entire skin area. It is not clear yet whether the neodymium laser, 10,600 Å is absorbed as effectively in the epidermis and dermal vessels, as is the ruby laser of equivalent energy density. In exit energies of neodymium laser in the order of magnitude of 200 joules, extensive surface charring is produced and some telangiectasia develops. In some uncontrolled experiments on the Caucasian skin of man, effects of the neodymium laser are less marked on the surface.

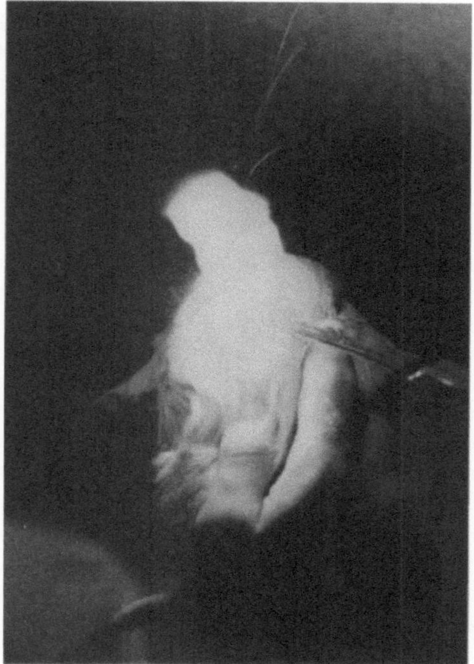

Fig. 18. Plume from impact white hair albino guinea pig. 100 joules exit energy pulsed ruby laser. Plume all from burned hair. No burn of underlying skin detected

In deeply pigmented tissues such as melanomas, the peripheral margins of the coagulation necrosis induced by the laser are sharply demarcated. In some melanomas, even with irregular extensions of the melanoma, the selective absorption of the laser is shown by the presence of the demarcation even at different depths in tissue.

When tissues do not possess intense pigments, efforts are made to try to color the tissue to try to increase energy absorption. This is done by dyes. These dyes may be applied topically, injected or given by perfusion into veins or arteries. The dyes are vital dyes, the non-toxic tissue colorants, and also the toxic dyes. The reason for the use of toxic dyes is that the cytotoxic properties of the dye moiety may have some synergestic effect on the laser reaction in living tissue. The dyes most commonly used in laser investigative work are suspensions of Indian Ink, Janus green, Evans blue, methylene blue brom phenol bleu (locally) and copper sulfate. In the study of the use of so-called specific tumor colorants, nile blue sulfate and malachite green are used.

When dyes are painted only on the surface of the tumor area, the laser impact will remove only the surface layer, often without very little damage to the under lying tissue. This can be shown by use of low energy lasers and the topical application to the skin of Indian ink. Topical dye absorption has been tried also with dimethyl sulfoxide (DMSO) as a vehicle. Even this effective vehicle does not produce too much absorption and penetration by the dye. Sometimes, the selective action of the laser may protect adjacent important structures as major vessels or nerves.

Injection of dye may make for a more uniform distribution. Efforts have been made to try to select the area of dye deposition by injecting it in a specific area or by the use of coated dye particles as suggested by LIEBERMAN. The impact of the laser destroys the dye coating so that it becomes much more diffuse in the selected depth. In this manner, the laser impact may be limited largely, not completely, to the zone of the dye depot. Dye pigments may also be tattooed into tumors.

Dyes may be injected intravenously. This is done especially with fluorescein and with investigative studies for brain tumors. Dyes may be injected into arteries. This perfusion will color tumor masses. To stain the blood vessels in the fundus of rabbits, MARTENS has injected methylene blue into the carotids. The cancer chemotherapist then has also been able to inject dyes intraarterially with perfusion techniques in order to saturate the tumor and provide for maximum absorption of the laser impact. The effectiveness of dye absorption can be studied by phase contrast microscopy and by a crude bio-assay technic by the observation of the effect of different impacts of the laser. The development of laser chemistry will determine whether the dye changes by the laser radiation still keep a vital dye safe for tissue. WILEY has indicated that after laser radiation of methylene blue, electron spin resonance signal may even be stronger for the next twenty-four hours. This indicates the development of free radical formation in the dye.

The whole subject of the selective dye absorption by tumors, especially tumors of the brain is under detailed in investigation by BROWN in our laboratory. As indicated previously, some of these dyes are vital staining and some are, also, cytotoxic in their own right. This property will increase the efficiency of the laser treatment. Such dye studies, then, will extend greatly the applications of laser surgery in the field of neurosurgery.

There is interest also as to whether dye absorption can be used for laser treatment of involved regional lymph glands. GILCHRIST has done studies on the suffusion of particles of ferrite, an iron oxide, into lymph glands, then their exposure to 100 KW generator for the production of hyperthermia (?). Dye particles can be absorbed by regional nodes or can be injected into regional nodes. Evans blue produces an extensive coloration of the tissue on local injection into a lumph gland. With multiple injections of a suspension of India ink, it is possible to color a small node. Then focused impacts of the laser may be given at different angles directly into the gland. As yet, there is not enough data to indicate the treatment areas and energy densities of ruby and neodymium laser required for complete coagulation necrosis of the gland. With metastatic glands of melanoma, it is often difficult to differentiate after laser impact between melanoblasts of the tumor and the reactive cells acting as phagocytes for the melanin.

It is obvious then, that the color of a tumor to be exposed to the laser is important. This color may be due to pigments normally present or added artificially. Vascularity of a lesion also is important as regards color quality. Vascularity indicates the total volume of blood vessels in the tumor target area of the laser, blood flow, oxygen content, the thickness and "character" of the blood vessel wall. This is of great importance in our studies on the laser treatment of angiomas. Some other features of tissue which contribute to its optical properties for laser treatment are collagen, ground substance, reticulum, amino acids, etc. These factors have been examined but little as regards absorption of the laser. It is obvious that continued research in color means advance in laser cancer research.

Chapter 5

Laser Radiation of Tissue Cultures

The laser head, attached to a microscope is a significant advance in instrumentation for cytology and cytogenetics. The laser beam may be focused by the optics so that the beam size can be reduced to a diameter as fine as one micron. This has been done by BESSIS. The laser beam may also impact microscopic preparations including tissue cultures through an arrangement outside of the microscope with the laser beam reflected into the microscope, yet the laser attacted to a microscope makes for greater technical control of laser microscopy. However, laser beams of other types of lasers such as Q-switching, second harmonics, gas lasers of various types, etc. may be directed from an external source through the microscope system. This flexible arrangement increases the range of laser microscopy.

The earliest developments in the field of laser microscopy were done by BESSIS. His basic studies of the impact of red cells and various protozoans provide significant as well as dramatic representations of the effect of the laser by time lapse cinematographic techniques. In these fascinating movies is seen the phagocytosis of the lased red cells by the energetic and aggressive white cells and in these studies also is seen the effect of the avoidance of the lased Euglena by the neighboring organisms. The influence of color by the addition of vital dyes to increase the absorption of laser impacts was also shown. SAKS ZUSOLO and KOPAC have used the laser head with the microscope for studies not only laser radiation, but combined with microsurgical techniques. They have studied ameoba and on the plant Nitella.

The most extensive studies in the field of laser cytology, including cytogenetics, have been done by ROUNDS and his associates at the Pasadena Foundation for Medical Research. In these techniques he has shown the significance of color in the absorption of laser radiation with studies of tissue cultures of pigmented retinal epithelium and melanoma. The pigmented cells show marked sensitivity to 6943 Å. The unpigmented cells were less sensitive to laser radiation except second harmonics. The real changes at cellular level of the absorption of laser radiation by unpigmented tissues were shown also by ROUNDS by studies on the changes in contracture of smooth muscle cells, rhythmic movements of heart muscle, ciliary movement. These studies indicate then, that there is some effect of the laser energy even on so-called transparent cells.

When blood is impacted by the laser, the red cells show significant change. White cells in the target area show very little gross change. However, if they are watched through microscopy they show changes in motility. FORRISTAL has also worked with changes in phagocytosis property of the white cells after the laser impact, and in studies of alkaline phosphatase. Biochemical studies have been done also by ROUNDS in tissue culture in relationship to adenosine triphosphate and also to diphosphopridine neucleotide.

The tissue culture techniques provide a technique for the testing of living cells for the production of abnormal cells from laser radiation. The testing can be done with biochemical investigations, essentially of DNA after laser radiation of cells or by the use of chromosomal analysis. The biological tests, as controls, for this type of experiment, could be free radical spectrometry after laser radiation. The test for chromosomal analysis would be similar to those used for testing of the effects of x-ray radiation on white cells in tissue culture.

Skin irradiated with laser has been cultured for chromosomal analysis. It is difficult to determine from cellular morphology whether the cells in tissue culture are fibroblasts or whether these are fusiform epidermal cells. Tissue culture techniques after laser radiation by SOUKUP and BLANEY have shown no abnormal chromosomes. Cultures of peripheral white cells after laser radiation of patients have been taken and subjected to chromosomal analysis and have shown no abnormal chromosomes. One tissue culture of vascular endothelium by ROUNDS and OKIGAKI have shown on the third subculture dicentrics and chromatid breaks. These studies are continuing. It is especially important that such studies be done in relationship to Q-switching techniques, because high peak power outputs have been suspected to produce Grenz rays. It is necessary that all these studies in cytogenetics should have adequate controls with other radiation modalities such as x-ray, Grenz ray, and ultraviolet radiation, radiation from the plasma of the plasma torch, and xenon light itself. Even in clinical investigative studies, the control factor of xenon light is often omitted. Yet, part of the incident beam on the target area may contain some of the xenon light from the xenon flash tubes of the laser head.

In the field of cytogenetics, the DNA metabolism in mammalian cells after laser radiation has been studied by ROUNDS and ADAMS. The DNA metabolism was detected by autoradiographic techniques following incubation of tritiated thymidine. Further development in the field of laser radiation will be the cytological and cytogenetic testing of the new lasers such as the argon laser, carbon dioxide laser and the like.

Of interest in cancer research is the combined use of x-ray radiation and cytotoxic agents with laser radiation in tissue cultures. These experiments have been initiated already in clinical cancer research with patients receiving gamma ray, yttrium, 90 nitrogen mustards, 5-FU in conjunction with laser radiation. The clinical studies are very difficult to control. It is obvious that controlled quantitatively equivalent sequences be done with either the laser radiation first and the other radiation modality second, or the use of the other radiation first, then the laser radiation. Then these same or different sequences have to be repeated with the use of cytotoxic drugs. All this complicates the radiation studies. It is the opinion of ROUNDS that x-ray and gamma radiation are synergistic in tissue culture techniques. It appears also that 5-FU and laser radiation may also be synergistic to tissue culture techniques of Hela cells. So, tissue culture may offer some significant information as to the synergistic effect of laser radiation with other forms of radiation and even with cytotoxic agents used in cancer chemotherapy.

Tissue culture techniques may be used also in the field of cancer research by studies of tissue cultures from the areas impacted with the laser compared with the areas which are not impacted with the laser. Such cultures can be examined for morphologic changes, continued growth or the development of any chromosome abnormalities, other than the chromosome abnormalities which the control area does show. Enzyme studies may also be done. The combination of the field of laser cytology and cytogenetics with immunoelectrophoresis may be of value in the immunobiological studies on tissues after laser impact.

The laser attached to the microscope can be used for studies of the effect of the laser on living blood vessels such as the mesoppendix of small animals. In these instances, the laser impact produces either thrombosis and hemorrhage or both. Initial studies in this dynamic field done by KOCHEN and his associates have been continued in other laboratories. Vascular anastomoses have been done by laser impact. The addition of dyes has been used to implement the studies of laser coagulation. These investigations are of importance in regard to the spreading factor of the effect of the laser by means of the thrombosis of the vessels in the target area.

Lasers attached to a microscope may be used for studies on the effect of cultures of bacteria and fungi. These cultures may be analyzed for pleomorphism, for the development of any type of abnormalities which can be continued. Such studies will aid in the studies of DNA on bacterial mutation.

The laser attached to microscope has also been used to impact the fertile chicken egg with selective areas of impact so that the development of congenital abnormalities can be observed grossly. This opens up an entire field of impaction of ova and even embryos for the selective action of the laser. The focusing of the beam through the microscope makes for delicate microsurgical manipulation with the laser. In the preparation of delicate miniature laboratory instrumentation, the microwelding and microdrilling by the laser microscope may be of help in the development of such micromanipulation instrumentation.

It is obvious then, that the laser microscope is an important instrument in the research laboratory, and will continue so, irrespective in the future of lack of clinical uses of the laser in cancer surgery.

Chapter 6

Laser Research in Cancer in Animals

In the investigation of the effect of the laser in cancer, research has proceeded in orderly stages. First there was basic research on laser radiation of tissue cultures and then the research on cancer in animals, and then the treatment of cancer in man. It must be remembered that unlike cancer research with gamma radiation, laser frequencies of lasers are in the visable and near-visable light ranges. Therefore, the reactions depend upon the optical systems in tissues which accept the laser beam. Studies on impact of the laser on cancers, not only in superficial tissues but also in the subcutaneous or deeper tissues of animals may offer different problems of light reflection, absorption, and transmission than in similar areas of man. The effect of coagulation necrosis induced by the laser may also have a different systemic response in animals than in man. Research with tumors transplanted into animals may also have a

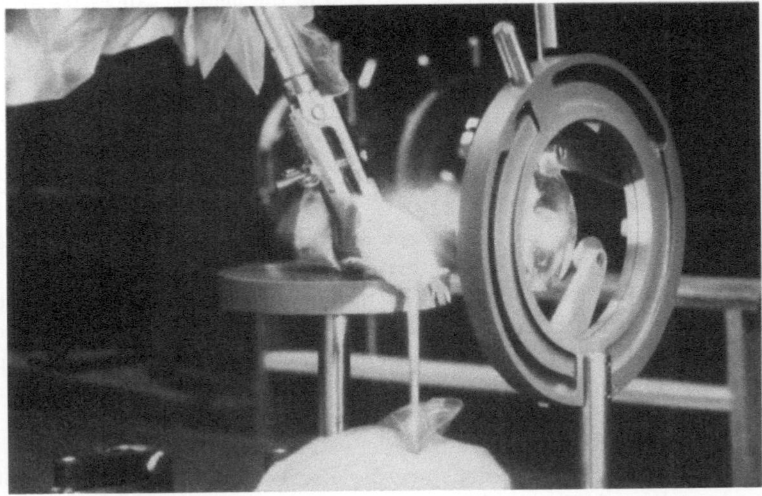

Fig. 19. Photograph of the technique of impact of white mouse with methylcholanthrene induced tumors by means of focussed beam of pulsed ruby laser

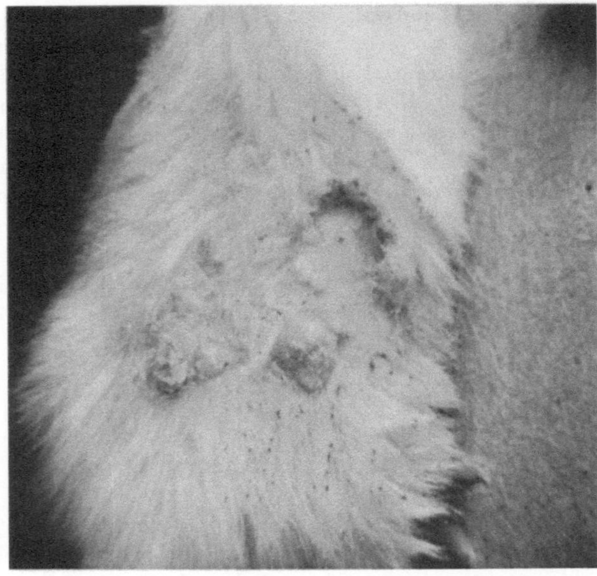

Fig. 20. White mouse showing only superficial charring of papillomatous methylcholanthrene tumors (Barich) after laser impact. 300 joules exit energy ruby laser

different immunologic response from those tumors which arise spontaneously in animals. These are but some of the restriction or limitations which must be considered in analysis of the results of laser treatment of tumors in animals.

In the United States, the basic studies of animal cancer have been done by McGuff, Klein and Fine, and Minton and Ketcham. Our laboratory has also

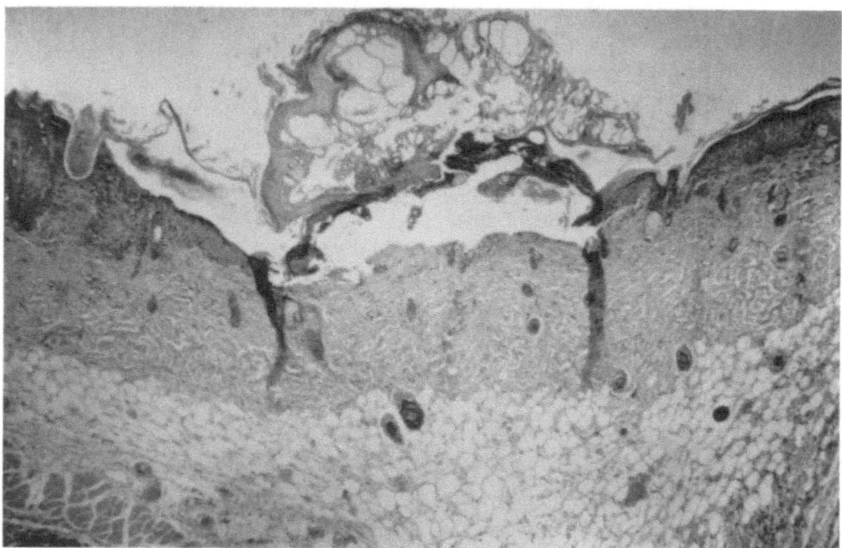

Fig. 21. Microscopic section showing skin section of white mouse with hyperkeratotic lesions induced by methylcholanthrene painting after high energy laser impact. 1200 joules exit energy pulsed ruby laser. There is surprisingly only superficial reaction in hyperkeratotic area and in epidermis, hematoxylin-eosin × 35

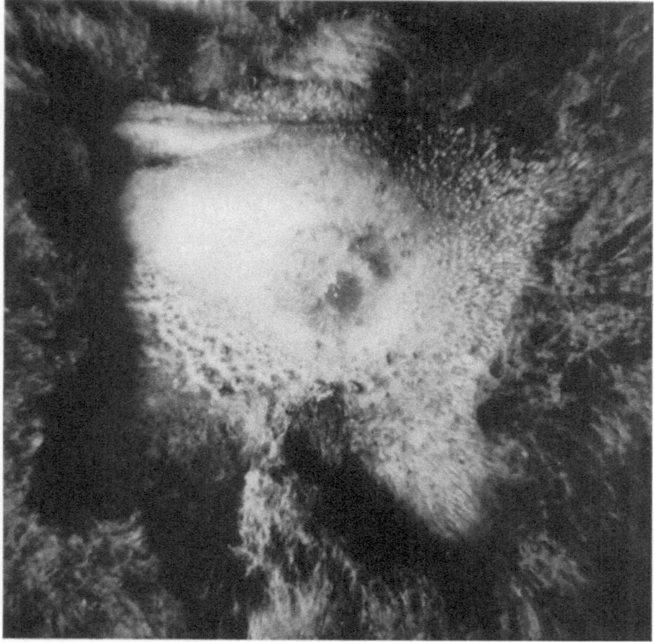

Fig. 22. Impact of laser on shaven area 4 days after inoculation polyoma virus (Sabin) in flank of hamster. 1200 joules exit energy ruby laser showing burning of hair, bleeding, superficial charring

studied laser treatment of tumors induced in animals and BROWN has initiated laser treatment of tumors of the nervous system.

Some of the tumors which have been studied in animals include:
1. Melanomas
   a. Pitt 41 melanoma implant
   b. Cloudman S-91 melanoma
   c. Harding-Passey melanoma
2. Carcinomas
   a. Lewis Bladder carcinoma C57-6
   b. human adenocarcinoma
   c. epidermoid carcinoma from methylcholanthrene
3. Sarcomas
   a. Ridgway Osteogenic sarcoma
   b. fibrosarcoma induced by methylcholanthrene
4. Miscellaneous tumors
   a. hepatomas in the Rhesus monkey
   b. polyoma virus tumors (SABIN).

Additional tumors continue to be added to this list.

The animals used for tumor studies include the Syrian hamster which McGUFF has used for cheek pouch inoculation and mouse strains which include the following: (1) the Swiss for the Harding-Passey melanoma and the Ridgway Osteogenic sarcoma, (2) the DBH-1 for the Cloudman S-91 melanoma, (3) C57-6 for the Lewis

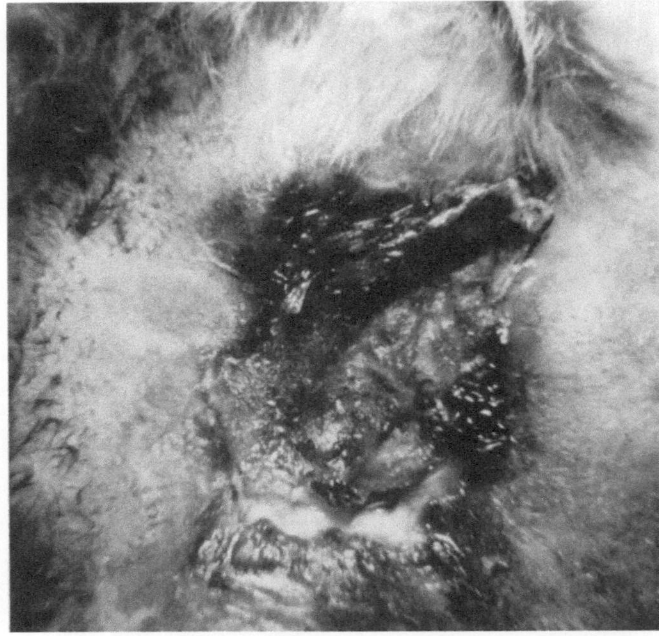

Fig. 23. 25 days after laser impact 1200 joules exit energy in polyoma virus induced tumor. There is central necrosis and continued extensive growth of tumor. Laser treatment had no effect and did not appear to accelerate tumor growth

bladder carcinoma, (4) CDBA-2Fl hybrid mouse for the Cloudman S-91 melanoma, (5) the hamster for the polyoma virus of Sabin, (6) the white rat for the methycholanthrene painting, and (7) Rhesus monkey for hepatomas.

In the inoculation experiments it is necessary that the hair be clipped or chemically epilated, since the hair will absorb a considerable mass of the laser radiation and deprive the tumor of this radiation. The cheek pouch technique of McGuff allows for maximum impact by the laser. Impacts and biopsies are done usually under light ether anesthesia or Nembutal. It is important that the Nembutal anesthesia be given carefully, otherwise the animals may die and long term studies be incomplete.

Animals presenting large or ulcerative lesions or lesions showing extensive coagulation necrosis should be kept in separate cages to avoid secondary trauma and infection and cannabalism by their cage mates.

In brief, the instrumentation used to treat the tumors has been the instrumentation available in laser technology. This includes (1) high and low energy pulsed ruby lasers, (2) the high and low energy pulsed neodymium lasers, (3) the Q-switched high peak power outputs of the ruby and neodymium laser, (4) the argon laser of 4 watts 4880—5215 Å, (5) the helium neon gas laser 6253 Å, (6) the nitrogen gas laser 3— 371 Å and (7) CO_2 laser 106,000 Å.

Laser impacts were given in calculated doses as unfocused, surface focused, and even as depth focused. Observation was recorded by gross inspection, by high speed picture techniques, which can show the fascinating plumes of the laser impact. High speed color photography shown by Minton of laser impact on a melanoma produces a picture resembling that of an atomic bomb mushroom cloud. Biopsies are taken at intervals after impact. The biopsy should be small enough and kept clean to avoid complicating the progress of the tumors. Biopsy controls are necessary, since scarring may obscure and conceal small deeply growing active tumor masses. As in the controlled studies of therapy routines of human cancer, it is often difficult to decide just where to take the biopsy. After the results of treatment have reached a plateau, then selective biopsies are taken, usually from the active areas as well as the areas which appeared to have improved.

Effect of laser treatment on animals maybe studied also by analyses of blood proteins and immunoelectrophoresis. The purpose of these studies is to determine the systemic effect of the laser impact, as well as attempts to initiate studies of the immunobiology of the laser induced tumor necrosis.

In the study of the reaction induced by the laser, it is also necessary to know the effect on the neighboring structures such as blood vessels, nerves, bone, etc. All this should be considered in the analysis of the progress of the local reaction. Cachexia developing in experimental animals may not only be the result of laser necrosis, but also necrosis of adjacent tissues and even of secondary infection or widespread metastases.

Controls, then, so necessary in experimental cancer research, must be observed also in the field of the application of the laser. It has been mentioned previously about the need for controls in regard to transplanted tumors and spontaneously developing tumors of animals. In transplantation experiments, control tumors must be available for observation. The technique of the inoculation of the hamster cheek pouch allows for ready observation of the control inoculation site. The factor of spontaneous resolution, often confusing in cancer research, can be observed with multiple lesions of some tumors.

There are also problems involved in attempts to study the various facets of the laser reaction in tissue. Admittedly, the chief interest in the laser is the thermal factor. Microminiature thermocouples with rapid response time may be used to study temperature changes if one realizes that this is the temperature of the heated tissue, not the laser impact temperature. In order to provide controls for thermal experiments, the use of the thermal cautery and the high frequency electrocoagulation must be considered. The difficulty, of course, is the attempt to develop controls comparative to the coagulation necrosis induced by the laser. For example, it is easy to simulate, on the surface, at least, similar charred areas of laser and of electrosurgery. The problem is to develop deep necrosis with the control characteristic of the laser. Therefore, with electrocoagulation, one goes deeper. At present we are using the plasma torch as a control for the thermal factor especially with the high output carbon dioxide lasers.

Too few experiments have been done in the attempts to control the sonic and ultrasonic factors of the laser impact with ultrasonic techniques of same intensities. This is also to be considered in the control experiments. Calibrated transducers maybe of help in these experiments.

For the so-called electromagnetic changes, gamma radiation, Grenz ray radiation, ultraviolet radiation, and even xenon light radiation must be considered as proper controls. It is difficult to develop comparative dosage schedules. How this theoretical concept can be realized in the actual experiment is not known, since too few of these controlled radiation experiments have been done. When there are multiple tumors in the same area of the same color quality surface and depth characteristic, then it is easier to do multiple controls. Untreated tumors must still be left as additional controls for all these modalities. It is obvious then that in certain circumstances, such as in experiments with hepatomas, it may be difficult in the same animal to have appropriate controls.

If controls are so difficult to set up in the radiation and thermal experiments, it is equally difficult to set up experiments to determine synergistic effects of the laser with x-ray, Grenz ray and with cancer chemotherapeutic agents. Here, save perhaps for x-ray and Grenz ray radiation, it is difficult to avoid systemic effects from the cancer chemotherapeutic agents, no matter how careful the topical applications of these materials. Cancer chemotherapeutic agents used in current cancer laser research include various nitrogen mustards, 5-fluorouracil, 5-desoxyuridine, 6-azuridine, podophyllin, and colchicine. Experiments then have to be done with all combinations of the laser and the chemical. With the difficulty of having constant standardized outputs of the laser especially in the high energy range, the problems are even more complicated. It is obvious at the present time, at least, that only generalizations may be made, not the presentations of specific quantitative data. At least these techniques will give some pilot ideas of attempts to develop an experimental system for this complex treatment routine for man.

From the preliminary studies of the past two years of laser therapy in animals and also in man, some data has been obtained. Some of the material is accepted; much of it is still controversial. However, one can generalize safely in a few areas. At least for high energy lasers, tumor necrosis may be induced in any type of tumor. The melanomas show the most significant intensity of tumor necrosis. To be most effective, the tumor must be accessible to the incident beam of the laser. It is obvious then, that tumors in the cheek pouch of the hamster may show a significantly greater effect of necrosis induced by the laser than a similar tumor of the same mass, same color qualities, deep in the flank. It may be necessary, then, that surgical intervention be required in order to make a tumor mass more accessible. This could refer, for example, to metastatic melanoma. Tumors deep in tissue may be reached only with doses focused deep into tissue. The depth of laser reaction can be observed only with controlled biopsy studies, not by surface observation of the target area of the impact.

The fibrosis induced by the laser impact is a non-specific type and may or may not be complete as regards persistency of tumor cords. Fibrosis often is relatively not completely resistant to laser impacts, even high energy.

Since the vascularity of the tumor also affects its response to the laser, the more vascular the tumor, usually the greater absorption of the laser beam in the target area at the surface or focused in depth. This is true of small angiomas of man. In experimental cancer work in animals, McGuff has found the opposite.

The smaller the tumor, the more certain the degree of destruction. Although with melanoma the necrosis appears to spread from the impact area, the mechanism of this progressive spreading is not known. In other tumors, especially non-pigmented ones, there will be no spreading and even successive impacts of adjacent areas may miss active tumor zones. This has been found, for example, in laser therapy of basal cell epithelioma of man. There is conflicting evidence also on laser therapy causing spread of the tumor.

Minton and Zelen have attempted to develop a formula for the calculated energy density needed per mass of tumor. They have also attempted to define a specific wave length for tumor destruction as determined by the honogenates of tumor subjected to analysis by the Beckman spectrophotomer. As higher and higher laser energies become available, it remains to be seen whether these specifications continue for specific types of tumors.

One important need is to determine the relative values of equivalent energy densities of the pulsed ruby and the neodymium laser, for example, in the therapy of the melanomas of animals. Minton and Ketcham indicate that the high energy neodymium is much more effective in the therapy of the melanoma than is the ruby laser. Whether this holds for other types of experimental tumors is certainly not known at present. McGuff has found the helium-neon gas laser to be effective to some extent, after prolonged exposure, in experimental fibrosarcoma. Hard tumors such as these as a rule show less response to laser than the so-called "soft-tumors". As yet, too little is known about the effect of the high energy output argon gas and carbon dioxide lasers. These are under study now.

In an effort to understand these confusing results, again data from laser radiation must include specific figures as the laser used its power and power density exit energy, its energy density, the lens system, and also the duration and character of the pulse. In our experience, a prolonged increase of the pulse duration will give different biological effects. Before any dogmatic conclusions can be given as to the relative merits of the ruby, the neodymium, the argon gas laser, carbon dioxide gas laser, and the Q-switching techniques over pulsed laser radiation, all of these will have to be considered in strictly controlled experiments. With present deficiencies of experience in this type of experimental program, as yet, it is not possible to produce definite recommendations for such cancer therapy. In an attempt to control the experiment more, in addition to the review of the laser output itself and its local effect on tissue, thermistors have been used to record the tissue temperature changes, to determine the differences between the thermal effects of the various lasers presumably with the same optical systems of the same tumors. As indicated, acting thermocouples have been put at the impact site at various depths away from the impact to measure at intervals after the impact. This has been done by McGuff and by Minton. In general, the temperature has been higher closer to the impact area. This is concerned with surface impact and very little work of this type has been done yet with focused impacts deep in the tissue. As with many of the fields of current laser research, this phase, too, requires more controls. It is confusing since the thermistors usually have a slow response time in relationship to the millisecond or even nanosecond impulse pulse of the laser impact and are unreliable because of resistance changes. Special fast recording thermocouples will have to be used to compensate for the delay in pulse time response. Moreover, it is often suspected that the probe in the target area may be impacted itself by the laser and that the temperature change may be that of the effect on the probe itself, since temperatures of 100° rises have been recorded by Minton in the target areas. Klein and Fine have coated the thermistors to reflect the light. In brief then, have the thermocouples indicated only general heating of tissue not the immediate temperature of the target?

Studies of the coagulated areas continue to be made. As indicated before, our laboratory has done tissue cultures both of the impacted and non-impacted areas to attempt to find morphologic, biochemical and chromosomal differences between the two areas. Also, as Rounds has suggested, an attempt has been made to determine whether the toxic materials are elaborated in the laser impact mass. This is studied by extraction of this area, and residue used on tissue cultures of melanoma. Studies have been made also on the differences in the identity of the antibody in the impacted areas as compared to thermal burn tissue and as compared to normal tissue of the same organ also being studied in our laboratory. Another study which offers much for the future is the implantation of the malignant tumors in the brain of animals by Brown and the controlled radiation studies of these in our laboratories with the various types of laser and with various types of tissue tumor colorants. Klein, Fine, Laor, Litwin, Donoghue and Simpson have studied the transplantation of Harding-Passey melanomas in mice after previous successful laser radiation of previously transplanted tissues. After laser radiation the second transplant failed to grow in five of six animals.

It is obvious then, that two factors in current laser research in cancer of animals are important. One is that investigative studies of laser radiation of tumor in animals is necessary and must be continued. Second, these very important studies should be continued by those familiar both with oncology and laser technology. Only in this way, with continued improvements in techniques, will there be valuable data available for the subsequent laser treatment of cancer in man. These studies in animals have already given us background for the application to man, but they should not rigidly limit our laser studies in man. It appears that in man high energy laser radiation is needed and in animals often laser radiation of low energy types is effective enough.

In brief, then, for tumors in animals, laser treatment may show minimal reactions, significant responses and even, according to KLEIN and FINE, occasionally acceleration of growth. It is obvious that such diverse responses depend on the laser and its many parameters and the type of tumor which is treated. Also, there maybe a relationship to the time interval between the implantation and the development of the tumor and the time when laser therapy was used. The localization, accessibility, color of the tumor, as regards intrinsic or extrinsic pigment, and vascularity are also important. The general condition of the animal and the intensity of the growth of the primary tumor and its metastases are additional factors complicating the response of the tumor to the laser.

There is also a need for more techniques to make the laser more flexible to reach inaccessible areas of animals, such as in the lungs, deep in the peritoneal cavity, behind the viscera. This means studies of transmission through special quartz rods and tubes, neodymium doped glass and special mirror arrangements as well as more controlled studies on focusing in depth in tissue.

If there is any concern about the carcinogenic property of the laser, this can be investigated easier in animals and in tissue cultures than in man. We have initiated studies to show the effect of repeated impact of small doses on the guinea pig, rabbit, and hamster, and over a long period of time, effective large single doses. These are done also with the impact of areas injected with Freund's adjuvant, and adjuvant 65, as well as controls with x-ray, Grenz ray, ultraviolet, and xenon light. Studies are done in these animals and in white rats, and in mice, and in the hairless mice. It is important that such studies be continued in order to determine the hazards of laser radiation as regards laser carcinogenesis.

Chapter 7

General Consideration of Laser Treatment of Cancer in Man

It is obvious that laser instrumentation must be modified to make it more flexible for cancer therapy. Outputs must remain constant and measures should be provided for constant monitoring of each output. The low energy output laser will continue to be used for experimental work in animals, in some melanomas of man and often in the field of laser neurosurgery. But in the clinical research field in cancer, high energy outputs will be needed. Recent developments in the production of high output flexible ruby and neodymium laser operating room equipment and in the production of high transmission curved tapered quartz rods are encouraging. Laser technology must provide effective, reliable and safe instrumentation. It has been remarked before that those in laser technology who have responsibilities usually are not as interested in the biomedical applications. Continued progress of laser cancer research and demonstration of value will assure continued interest and development of laser surgery.

As usual in cancer research, data collected must be of sufficient detail and standardization of terminology so that it can be made easily available and understandable to other laser research groups. This means the adoption of standards of laser radiation by reference to those standards which are available in physics today. There must be included in the description of dosage and listing of laser used, power and power densities, the exit energies, peak, energy densities, lens system, target area, duration and character of the pulse. Although it may seem cumbersome in the present techniques, the listing of all these deails is necessary. In his manner, those in cancer research would be able to repeat or modify the results of others.

When one has to consider instrumentation for increased flexibility to reach the depth in tissue, or to reach inaccessible areas or into cavities, more research must be done with such optical systems which can transmit or reflect the laser beam. These are prisms, mirrors (gold and silver plated especially), quartz tubes, quartz rods and other optical instrumentation. The properties of the beam transmitted or reflected from these areas must be known as regards coherency and energy loss. It is not certain as yet whether coherency is necessary for biomedical research although coherency is necessary for accurate focussing and for laser holography.

Progress in gas laser has been significant recently so that now high output instruments are available for cancer research. These include the argon, a carbon dioxide and ultraviolet lasers. For work in highly vascularized organs such as the liver, the argon laser may be used. As progress in the development of junction diode lasers continues, this type of laser may be able to be used for cancer research. Low output requirements for work at very low temperatures limit the value of this. This type of laser has great possibilities as regards efficiency, miniaturization and consequent great flexibility, etc.

The development of laser transillumination may offer some help in the field of cancer diagnosis not as valuable as that of infrared mammography or even soft tissue x-ray photography at the present time. Investigations are being done to determine, whether laser transiluminography is without any effect on tissue. Laser photography, and third dimensional laser holography are being developed in detail. This may also offer some value for cancer diagnosis, for cancer teaching and for scientific exhibits.

The type of tissue responses in laser radiation must be investigated to determine if there are any significant differences from those which are produced through other methods of cancer treatment. The multiple facets of the laser reaction in tissue of thermal, pressure, sonic, electromagnetic types offer considerable challenge to the pathologist in the interpretation of dynamic pathology. Even though vascular surgery is being done by laser as to produce anastomoses, and with the argon laser to arrest hemorrhage, little is known about the effects of the prolonged laser radiation of the blood. Immediate vascular reactions to the laser include hemorrhage, thrombosis and subsequent embolic phenomena.

Fiber optics offer another opportunity for further development of laser instrumentation. As yet, fiber optics do not permit transmission of significant energies of laser. Fibers doped with neodymium may correct this. However, fiber optics may transmit high output argon laser beams.

It is obvious also that one cannot continue laser research without biochemical studies of the effect of the laser on the cells. One of the phases in this is the study of free radical formation as determined by electron spin resonance spectrometry. The laser cancer treatment of man should be followed by biochemical studies of effects on enzymes. Elastic ultra-sonic and retoil pressure waves bring the new field of sonochemistry into laser research.

For the immunobiology of cancer, the laser beam offers another opportunity to study cancer changed by the laser impact. DNA may be affected by production of second harmonics in tissue from the impact of the laser beam on amino acids. Investigative studies include lasers in combination with gamma ray, Grenz rays and cancer chemotherapeutic agents.

For the cancer surgeon, the two essential problems of the laser for the immediate future are simple. These are — is the laser treatment effective and is it safe? In order to determine whether this is effective or not, the experienced cancer surgeon must include laser instrumentation in the operating room. He must learn about lasers, must know how to use them and must fit them in his program as they are needed. He alone can determine what the future of the laser will be in the field of cancer. Again, this is not another exercise in radiobiology but just a new type of instrument for the surgeon. We like to call this an "optical knife", precise, powerful. It is, however, the surgeon who will determine whether these attributes are warranted. In the past, the surgeon has had various teams. Now he must become acquainted with physicists and engineers. They must look over his shoulder even in the sterile fields of the operating room, otherwise the surgeon may become confused and disturbed and discard something which has great potential value.

In medical centers, surgeons must be assigned to evaluate laser surgery. Departments of engineering and physics provide the initial stimulus for laser research.

Unfortunately the public has been subjected to flights into fantasy projected by the flashings of the laser beam. This has forced even the calm investigator to expect immediate miracles.

In brief, in cancer research, studies with the laser must continue.

Chapter 8
Laser Treatment of Melanomas

Because the studies in our laboratory and the work of other investigators of the effect of color on the absorption of the laser energy, patients with melanomas early in the course of our clinical investigative studies were treated. The initial experiments

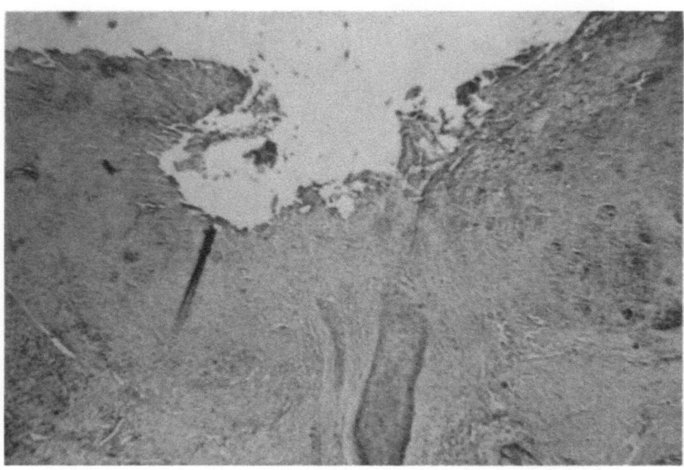

Fig. 24. Excision of melanoma upper back 24 hours after laser impact 50 joules exit energy laser showing deep coagulation necrosis sharply demarcated with relative resistance of the hair follicle. Hematoxylin-eosin × 50

were done by impacts of the laser of freshly excised deeply pigmented melanoma tissue. In addition, cytological material from ulcerative melanomas was exposed to unfocussed laser beams of low energy laser impact of 0.2—0.5 joules and the selective destruction of the melanoma tumor cells was found.

The first patient in a clinical series treated in 1962 was in reality a deeply pigmented angiokeratoma. The diagnosis was not made until excision biopsy after the

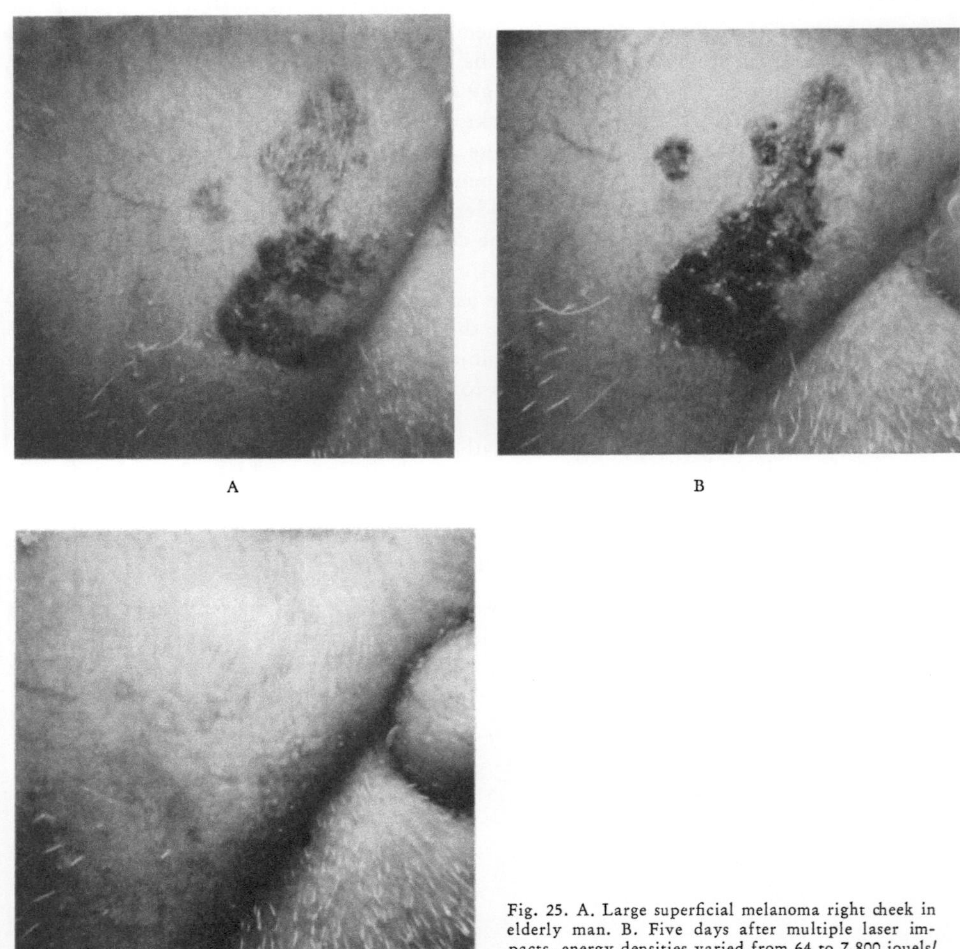

Fig. 25. A. Large superficial melanoma right cheek in elderly man. B. Five days after multiple laser impacts, energy densities varied from 64 to 7,800 jouels/cm². C. One year after laser impacts — biopsies negative

laser impact with 50 joules/cm² energy density. Only superficial changes were produced in this deeply pigmented lesion above the right knee. The next patient was a young man with a melanoma of the upper back. After biopsy, a small area was impacted with unfocussed ruby laser beam exit energy of 65 joules. This lesion was then excised widely after 48 hours. Detailed microscopic examinations were made. The significant histologic changes, previously reported, included sharp demarcation of the laser impact in the melanoma tissue and fairly deep extension of the coagulation necrosis. One feature of the section was the relative resistance of the pilosebaceous unit in the midst of the laser necrosis. This relative resistance of the hair follicle was

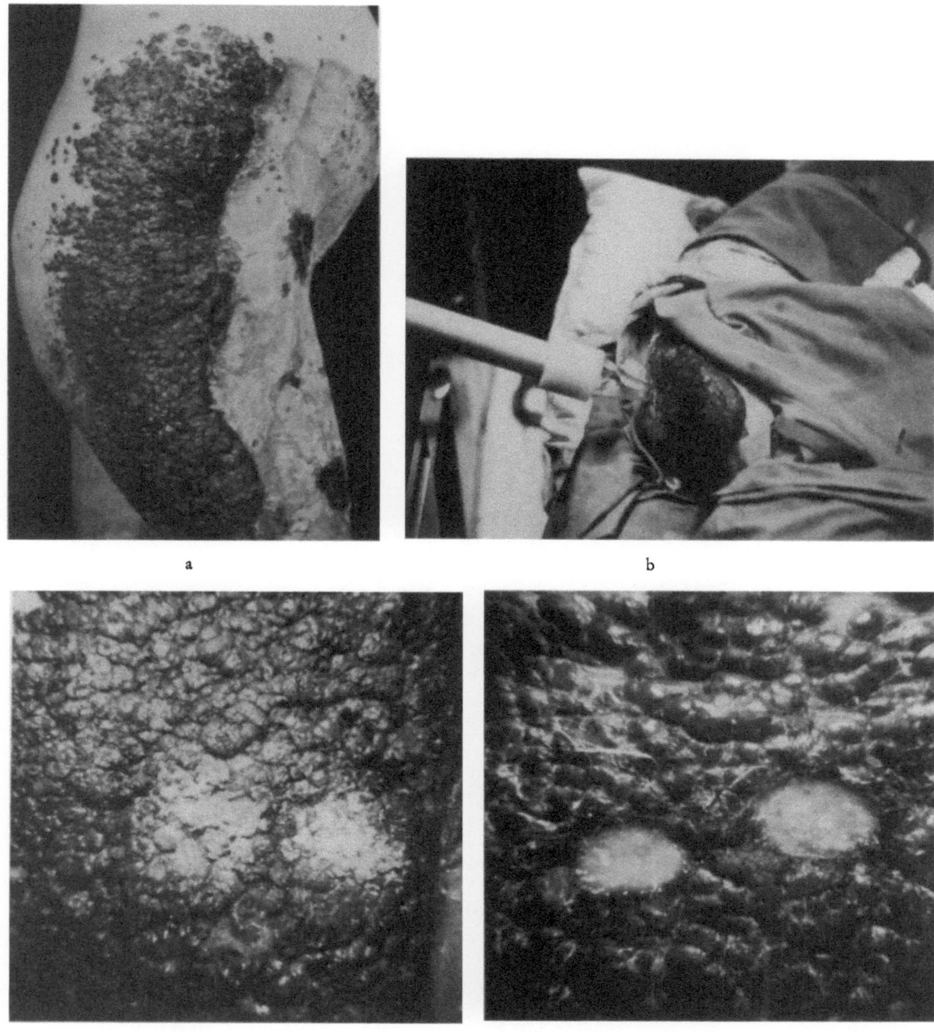

Fig. 26. a—d. Metastatic melanoma following excision of melanoma right thigh and skinning operation (Walter Reed General Hospital). b. Showing technique of laser treatment of small area with high energy laboratory model neodymium laser (Eastman) unfocussed beam exit energy 1160 joules. c. After impacts of 1160 joules unfocussed beam. d. Five days after impacts showing deep white necrotic areas

found also in later experiments on the skin of a patient. This is of interest in view of the recent investigations by KLEIN and his associates on the persistent depigmentation produced by the laser on hairs adjacent to the target area in pigmented skin of animals.

3*

Among the initial experiments of laser treatment of melanomas were those done by HELSPER on cutaneous nodules of metastatic melanoma. The nodules were exposed, impacted with the laser and then the incisions were closed. Controls included other modalities of therapy. The progress of these nodules was watched and significant progressive spread of necrosis was found in the nodules at intervals after laser radiation. There was also considerable phagocytosis of melanin pigment. This progressive necrosis of the melanoma after laser impact collaborated the early animal experiments of McGUFF, KLEIN, and FINE. McGUFF also used the laser radiation in cutaneous metastatic melanoma.

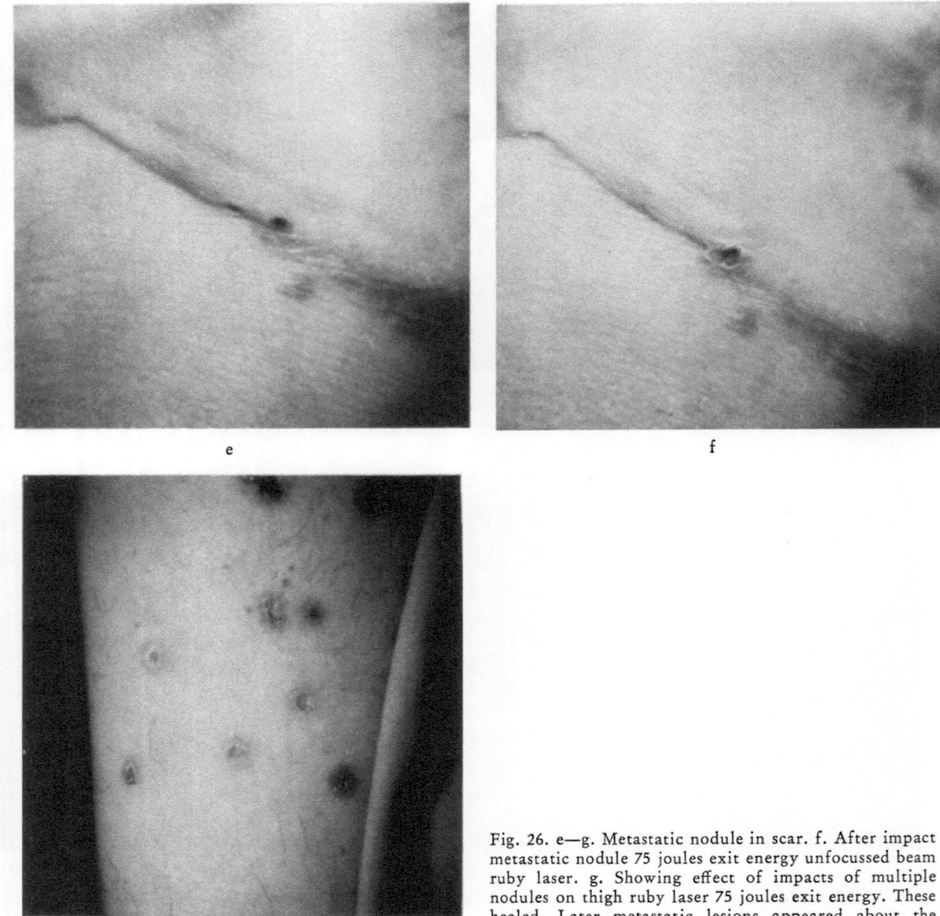

Fig. 26. e—g. Metastatic nodule in scar. f. After impact metastatic nodule 75 joules exit energy unfocussed beam ruby laser. g. Showing effect of impacts of multiple nodules on thigh ruby laser 75 joules exit energy. These healed. Later metastatic lesions appeared about the periphery of some

With the increasing availability of higher output of lasers, our investigations continued on clinical studies of the laser impact of melanoma. An extensive superficial melanoma of the cheek was treated with laser impacts. The dosage varied from 64 to 7,800 joules/cm², unfocussed and focussed. The patient was followed for one year later with multiple biopsies of the site. These were all negative. Death occurred from an intercurrent kidney infection. At autopsy, no evidence of metastatic melanoma in the viscera or skin was found. Additional patients studied in the laboratory included a middle aged woman with hundreds of metastatic skin nodules recurrent after radical excision and skinning operation for a recurrent melanoma of the mid-thigh. This patient was treated with ruby and neodymium laser — ruby laser 300 joules exit energy, neodymium laser (the special laboratory model of the Eastman Kodak neodymium laser) 1160 joules exit energy — and 1680 joules focussed 2 cm. depth in tissue. Seven months follow-up of this patient showed significant reactions following multiple laser impacts of many of the lesions. The 2 cm. focussed impacts produced a deep necrosis within five days with disappearance of all the black color of the melanoma in the target area. During a brief period of observations these became white. The small metastatic lesions showed initial clearing with later invasion from adjacent melanoma. The patient received also injections of autogenous extract of her melanoma in saline in complete Freund's adjuvant and also autogenous extract mixed in adjuvant 65. One year after laser impact there was still significant whitening of the laser areas. Recent examination of this patient has shown persistent scarring of laser treated areas, now with negative biopsies. There has been spon-

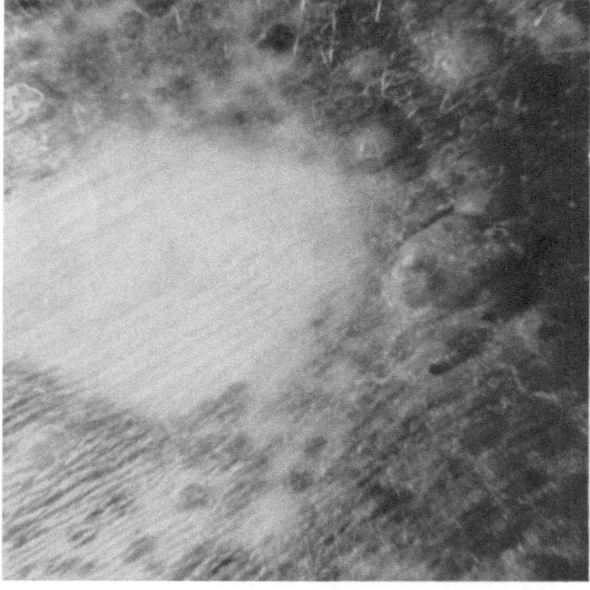

h

Fig. 26. h. 7 months after laser impact showing persistent white, smooth soft scar with biopsies negative for melanoma

taneous disappearance of many lesions with only dermal melanosis remaining. In addition, there has been an extensive fibroblastic response in untreated as well as in treated lesions. Detailed immunologic investigations by BLANEY and ROTTE in our Laboratory of Cancer Immunology have shown only negative data. The mechanism of her spontaneous responses and her fibroblastic reactions are unknown. Both laser treatments and her injections of autogenous extracts in adjuvant 65 are continuing. Recently, new distant nodules and pulmonary and bone metastases have appeared.

Additional patients included two patients with deep nodular masses in the neck. These on biopsy showed melanoma. The origin of these masses was unknown. In one

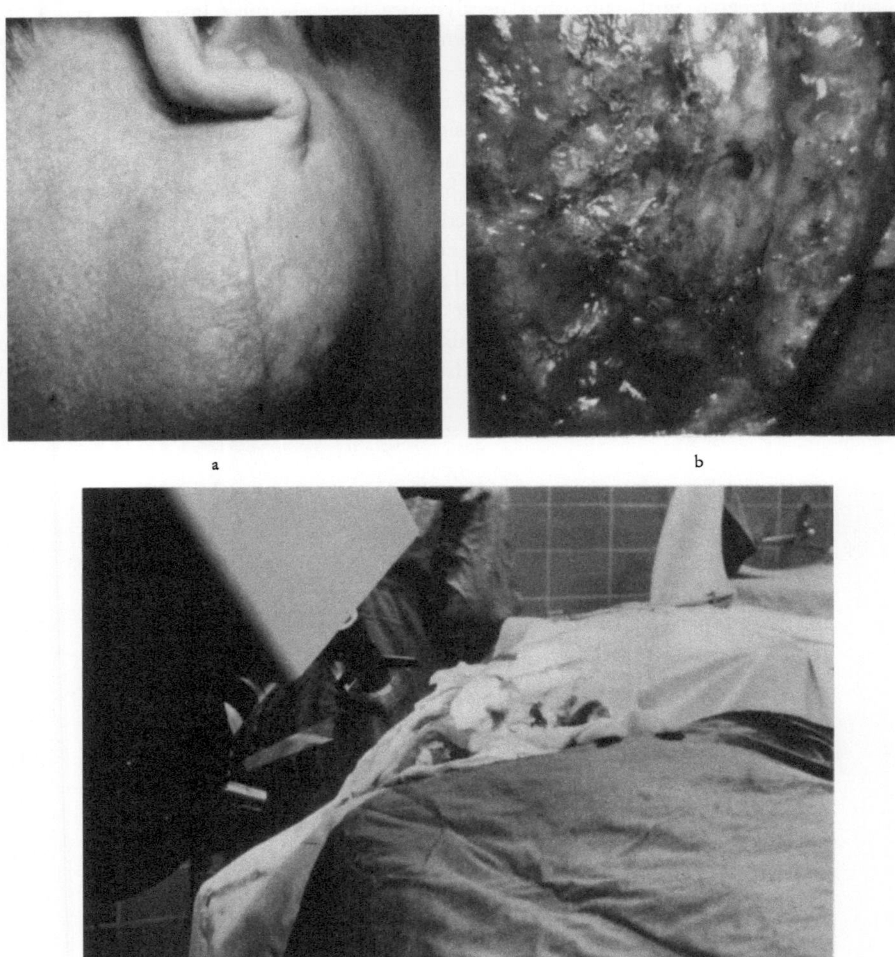

Fig. 27. a—c. Deep melanoma of neck 5 years duration. No evidence of visceral metastases. b. Exposure of tumor in operating room by Dr. V. E. SILER and multiple impacts, unfocussed, surface focussed and two centimeter deep focussed impacts through scar tissue covering. Only superficial necrosis developed but tumor mass became smaller. c. Second exposure after one year by Dr. V. E. SILER showing operating room set up with operating room ruby laser, 70 joules exit energy

patient, this had been present for some five years without any evidence of metastases. In the other patient, there was a small metastatic nodule in the axilla. These lesions, in both of these patients, were exposed in the operating room by Dr. V. E. Siler, Director of Laser Surgery at the Laser Laboratory. In the other patient, surgical exposure revealed deep masses of melanoma about the major vessels in the neck.

Multiple laser impacts, focussed and unfocussed, were given to the exposed tissues even to pigmented masses deep in the neck. The patients withstood the operations very well and during the brief period of observation, there were no significant reactions. Both patients were given in addition autogenous extracts of melanoma in complete Freund's adjuvant and adjuvant 65. In only follow-up of one year the lesions in both patients are not progressive. As yet, there are no visceral metastases in the laser impact area but there is are spread about the periphery.

Recently, in our laboratory BROWN and HENDERSON used an argon laser on loan from Bell Telephone Laboratories to excise a deep metastatic melanoma nodule in the tissue about the hip. Control studies on other subcutaneous nodules in this patient included high output neodymium laser 950 joules exit energy, on loan from Eastman Kodak, with direct impact through intact skin, ruby laser 200 joules exit energy transmitted through curved tapered quartz rods; and electrosurgery. Only

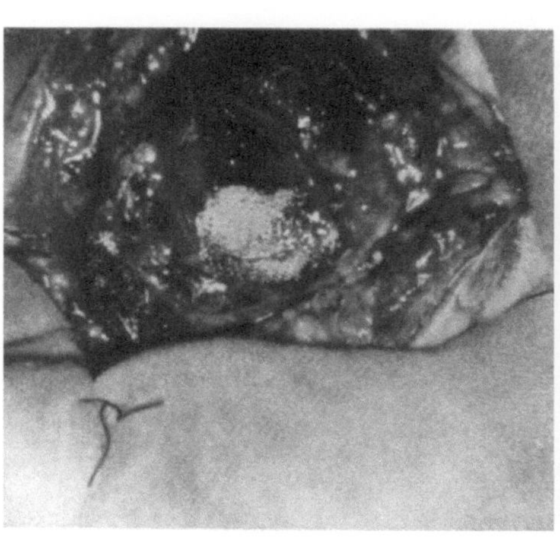 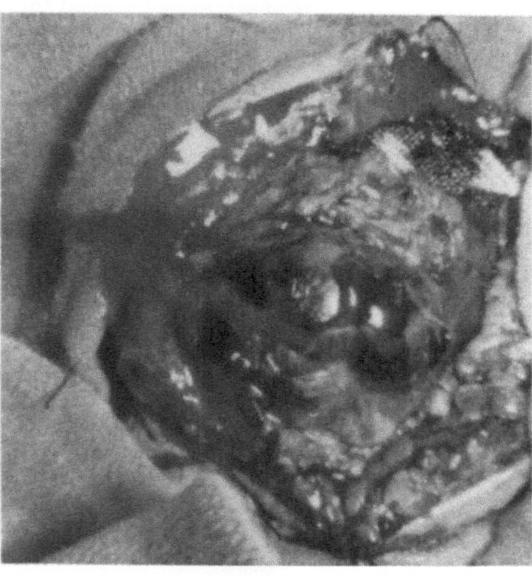

de

Fig. 27. d—e. Melanoma with fibrous tissue coverings dissected away. e. After 27 treatments — 7 focussed 3 cms. in depth and 20 unfocussed surface impacts

immediate follow-up studies are available. Responses to argon and neodymium laser were good with disappearance of the treated nodules. The carbon dioxide laser was used on an excised nodule to study the extent of the thermal reaction.

From preliminary experiments, it appears that the laser treatment should be considered as an investigative therapy in inoperable melanoma. The color quality of the pigmented melanoma insures absorption of the laser energy if the tumor is accessible to the laser. High energies are needed in deep masses, at least, 2—5000 joules/cm². In animal experimentations, it appears as if the neodymium high energy lasers are as effective as the ruby. In our experiments, with the high energy neodymium laser with 1160 joules exit energy, effective destruction and deep destruction of the melanoma were observed. With the improvement in technique, especially in the operating room, and with development of intraabdominal laser surgery, laser treatment may be given for visceral metastases. KETCHAM has established a program recently for the laser treatment of intrathoracic melanoma in the specially equipped laser surgical operating room of the National Cancer Institute.

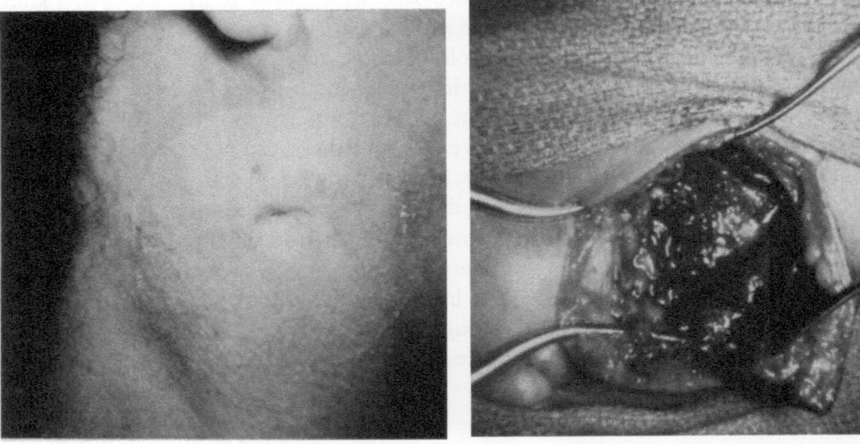

a　　　　　　　　　　　　　　　　b

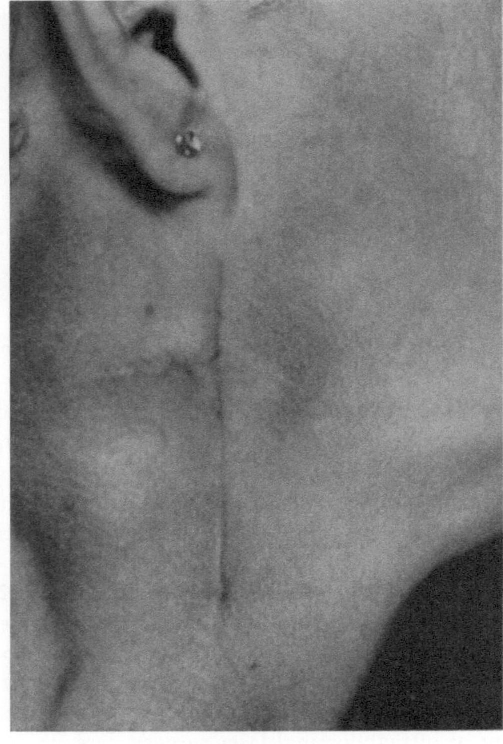

c

Fig. 28. a. Deep melanoma of the neck, recent duration. b. After exposure in operation room by Dr. V. E. SILER for laser treatment. c. Four months after laser treatment with reduction in size of mass. Later, new nodules developed in posterior area of mass

Some lesions of melanoma appear to show progressive changes in coagulation necrosis induced by the laser and spread far beyond the target area. The mechanism of this is not clear, as yet, (vascular thromboses, multiple absorptions, reflection, ultrasonic, and immunobiologic ?) but is obviously of definite therapeutic value.

In one patient, a recurrent melanoma of the scalp had metastasized to the diploe of the calvarium and was recurrent after a craniectomy. This patient was operated on by Dr. Robert McLaurin and Dr. Thomas Brown, of the Division of Laser Neurosurgery of the Laboratory. After extensive craniectomy and biopsies of the dura showing active melanoma, the edges of the wound were impacted with 80 impacts of laser through a curved quartz rod 70 joules exit energy, all entirely around the operative wound. Subsequent follow-up studies will determine the value of this in the prevention of recurrence of the melanoma in the diploe and adjacent tissues. With the

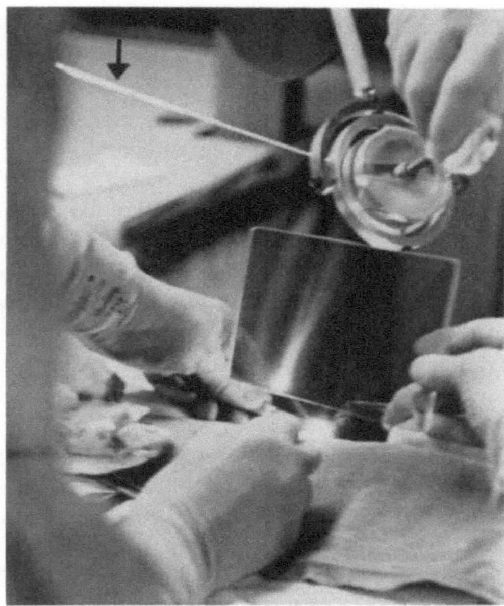

Fig. 29. Showing use of experimental argon laser, 2-watt output, on loan from Bell Telephone Laboratories, Inc., CW laser for excision of subcutaneous metastatic nodule of melanoma. This continuous-wave laser functions as a bloodles optical knife with the continuous beam reflected by mirror around the melanoma. Amber plastic screen is for eye protection of the operating surgeon from the intense fluorescence of the impact of the argon laser on the melanoma

high energy outputs used in this area, the safety of the laser for operations near the brain was demonstrated.

It is too early in the course of the investigations to determine the synergistic value of the laser and the chemotherapeutic agents such as Methotrexate, 5-Fluorouracil, nitrogen mustards, etc. in the therapy of melanomas. We have used these chemotherapeutic agents locally and systemically in patients receiving laser treatments. Methotrexate has especially been used in one patient who had received laser therapy. It was not possible to evaluate this combined therapy.

Melanoma is always a capricious reactor and the immunobiologic factor in this form of cancer is often of considerable interest and even of significance and always puzzling. The effect of the laser on immunobiology of the melanoma is not known. The experiments of KLEIN and FINE showing the resistance to melanoma re-innoculation of laser treated animals are of interest.

The initial results, then, in laser treatment of melanoma are encouraging enough to warrant continued investigative studies. This appears to be of value expecially in superficial melanoma where surgery cannot be done satisfactory and also in inoperable melanoma with accessible metastases.

Chapter 9

The Treatment of Epitheliomas

Epitheliomas which are multiple and accessible lend themselves readily to laser treatment. These lesions include chiefly pigmented and non-pigmented basal cell epitheliomas, squamous cell carcinomas both superficial and invasive. To enable the epitheliomas to absorb more laser energy, non-pigmented lesions have been colored with Evan's blue, Janus green, India ink in dimethyl sulfoxide (DMSO), and by copper iontophoresis and by tattooing.

Multiple lesions in the same patient afford opportunity for detailed control studies with different forms of treatment. For multiple basal cell epitheliomas such controls to laser therapy would include excision, curettement, electrosurgery, heat applications, controlled chemosurgery by Mohs' technique, Grenz ray,and x-ray radiation. Progress can be followed by thin section biopsy techniques. Unless the laser treatment offers any significant advantage over the other forms of treatment, there would be no practical need for this new investigative modality. Again, long continued observation with biopsy studies is needed to detect recurrences.

The follow-up is not as simple as it seems, because there is often a delayed response to laser treatment. In some instances, a biopsy shows very little necrosis in three weeks to a month after treatment, and then the response may develop. Subsequent biopsies then show complete disappearance. The fibrosis is not specific in type.

As usual, sclerodermic basal cell carcinoma is particularly difficult. Heavy fibrous masses may conceal active cords of basal cell epitheliomas for long periods of time until they reach the surface and become obvious. In one patient in our series of these basal epitheliomas, nodules in this patient proved on repeated biopsies to be simply cicatrix. However, later surgical excision by Dr. V. E. SILER showed tumor cords under deep cicatrix. It is emphasized that punch biopsies or biopsies of small areas cannot be used to follow the progress of a lesion, since that biopsy may represent only a part of a small area of the entire treated tumor mass. With small biopsies by razor blade technique, small narrow, deep biopsies may offer more significant information than the punch biopsy and will not interfere with the clinical observation in the post treatment. Unless the patient can be followed for prolonged periods of time and unless control studies can be done, these sclerodermic or morphoric or scarring basal epitheliomas should not be treated at present.

Some areas have been of special significance for laser treatment. These are basal cell epitheliomas of the tip of the nose and basal cell epitheliomas developing on extensive radio-dermatitis of the face. In these cases, the laser treatment has produced significant cosmetic results with the superficial types of lesions. For areas about the nose, ears, and near the eyes, quartz rods transmitting significant energy levels, as much as 1000 joules/cm² of energy density have been used. Impacts must be done carefully to avoid "skip" areas. Studies of shock waves are under way in our laboratory in regard to laser therapy of epitheliomas involving the external auditory meatus.

We have treated and have used pulsed ruby laser and neodymium laser for epitheliomas. The problem of adequate therapy appears to be adequate energy density and an adequate treatment or target area. In diffusely infiltrating ill-defined lesions, this has not been any easier than it is to treat these lesions with other modalities of radiation. The energy densities required depend upon the degree of infiltration, the

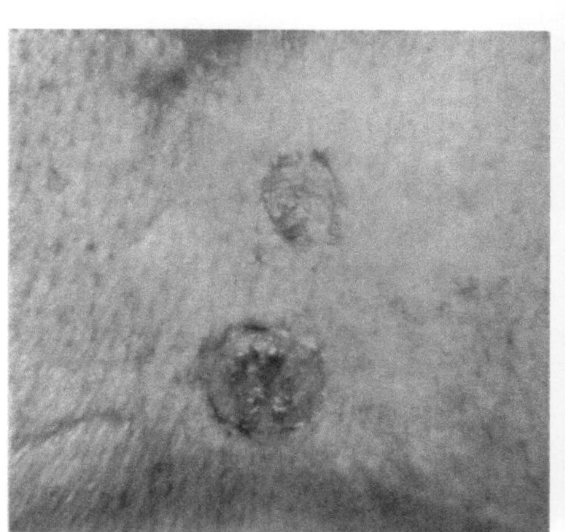
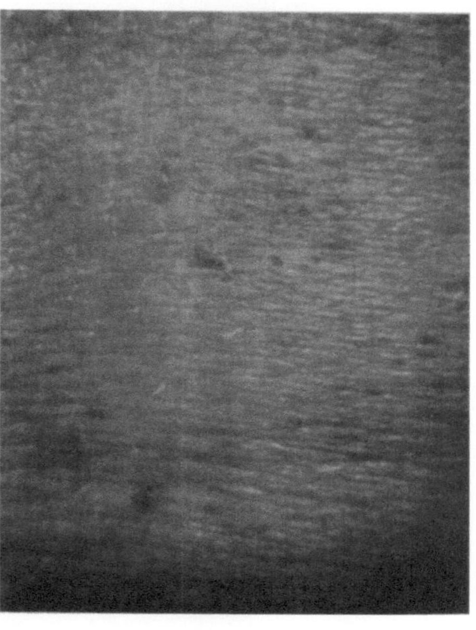

a   b

Fig. 30. a. Superficial basal epitheliomas of the lower back, lower lesion pigmented. b. Follow-up after one year — showing no obvious scarring

degree of pigmentation, and the fibrosis present. Whereas in other areas, as for example in laser eye surgery, one can go from the minimal to the maximal dose. This cannot be done for epitheliomas, for the first treatment of the epithelioma is important and the responsibility, as usual, for the adequate treatment of epitheliomas is with the first one who treats these lesions. Therefore, initially there must be adequate energy densities. Each case must be treated individually. Multiple impacts ought to cover the entire area with the so-called "adequate border around". If both focused and unfocused treatments are given, the focused treatments should be given first, since unfocused impact chars the surface and may interfere with subsequent treatments in depth. Unfocused surface impacts demand usually 75—100 joules/cm²; focused impacts demand 2000—3000 joules/cm². In the treatment of relatively broad areas, one must be careful not to miss any of the areas with multiple treatments. As yet, it is not possible to indicate the relative values of neodymium and ruby lasers. In the neodymium series for superficial epithelioma, we have used 200 joules exit energy of the pulsed neodymium laser. Treatments with the neodymium laser have often been unfocused to test the greater penetrating quality of the neodymium laser.

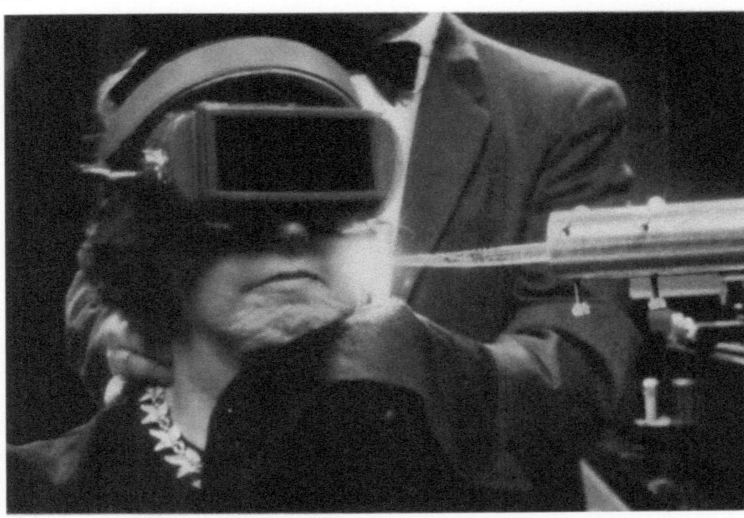

a

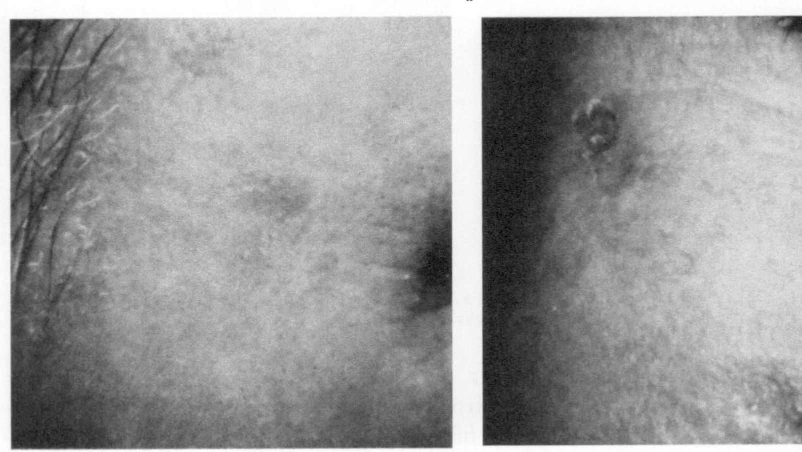

b   c

Fig. 31. a—c. Laser treatment of multiple basal epitheliomas of the face associated with x-ray dermatitis. Laser transmission through high quality quartz rods with energy densities 539 joules/cm². Accurate placement of beam is possible with such rods. b. Biopsy positive basal epitheliomas. c. After laser treatment

Since the laser therapy of the epithelioma has been given for only four years, it is difficult to critically analyze follow-up data. As we have reported from our Laboratory, failures have been due to inadequate treatment on the surface as well as in depth. In our experience, the recurrences have appeared about the periphery. In these failures it was assumeed that inadequate coverage of the lesion had been done. At present we are using frozen sections after laser treatment to check the extent of the reaction. To date, the lesions have shown none of the atrophic, telangiectastic scars such as are observed after x-ray radiation.

As indicated, the pathology of the laser radiation treatment is that of non-specific fibrosis. In the follow-up biopsies of the basal cell epithelioma, we have not

Fig. 31. d. Follow-up studies   d

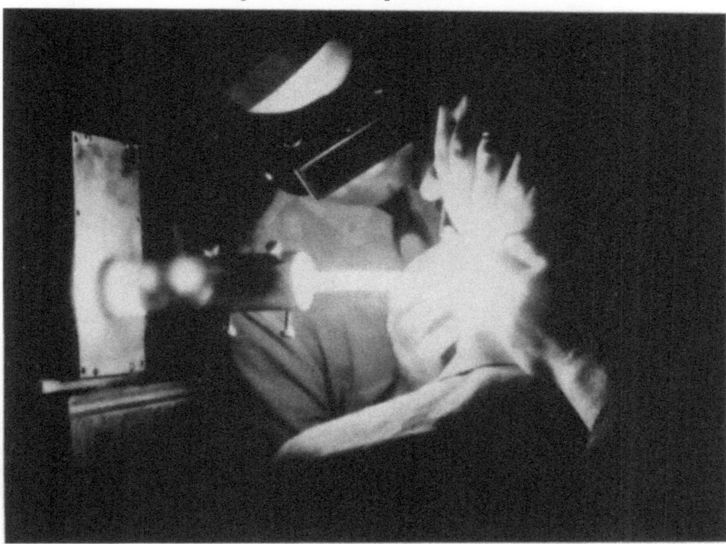

Fig. 32. Laser treatment of basal epithelioma of ear with curved quartz rod. Black and white copy of Ektachrome Infrared (Eastman) of impact. Later, recurrence at lower border.

observed the relative sparing of the pilosebaceous unit. This is not similar to that which has been observed in the follow-up studies on laser treatment of melanoma.

The treatment of squamous cell epithelioma has included recurrent inoperable squamous carcinoma of the thigh Bowen's disease, Paget's disease, and early invasive, so-called grade 1 and grade 2 squamous cell epithelioma. Again, the need for adequate surface carries coverage of the lesion, so-called adequate target area, and adequate energy density, has been shown until more knowledge of the effect of lasers on epitheliomas is available. The treatment with Bowen's has been satisfactory if the entire surface is radiated. The treatment of Paget's has been only investigative, since our studies were done on extra-mammary lesions as an investigative procedure prior to complete surgical excision.

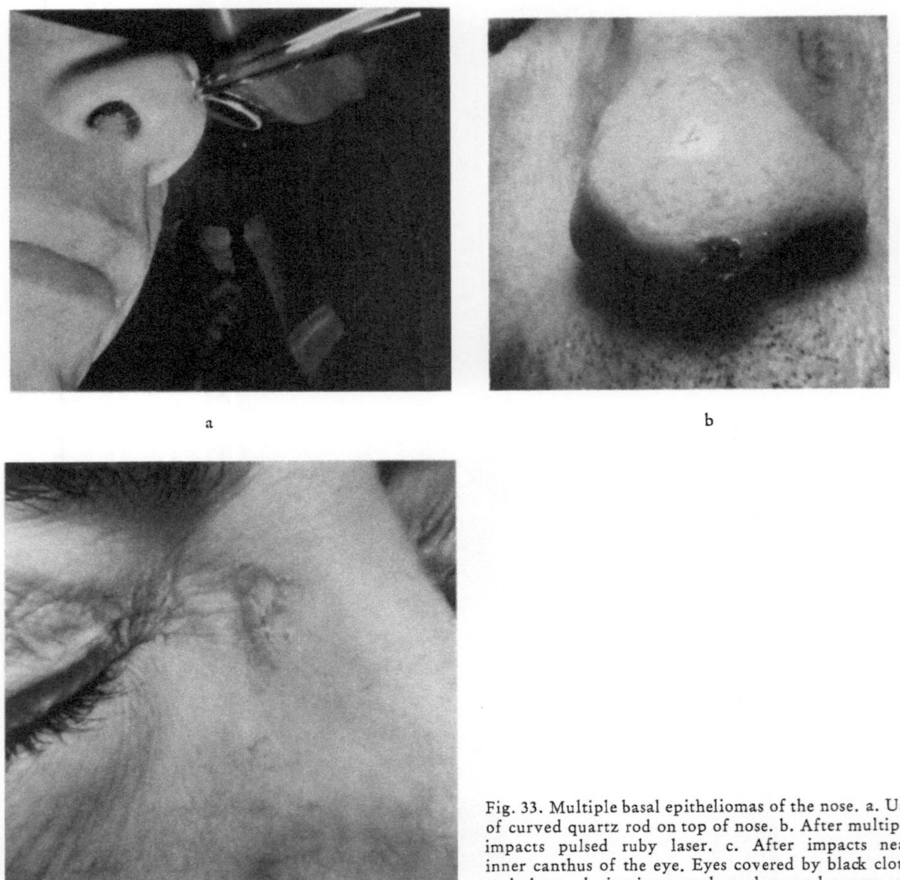

Fig. 33. Multiple basal epitheliomas of the nose. a. Use of curved quartz rod on top of nose. b. After multiple impacts pulsed ruby laser. c. After impacts near inner canthus of the eye. Eyes covered by black cloth and glasses during impacts through curved quartz rod resting directly on target

Experiments have been done on leukoplakia of the lips alone and after painting with Evan's blue and after injection of Evan's blue. The results of these preliminary studies show superficial coagulation necrosis. Detailed follow-up are as yet not available to indicate whether this therapy is superior to electro-surgery or not.

Laser treatment then, for accessible epitheliomas is but another area for current investigative studies. Not only is actual therapy of the lesions done, but it is possible to pursue investigative studies as to the mechanism of the action of the laser in these tumors.

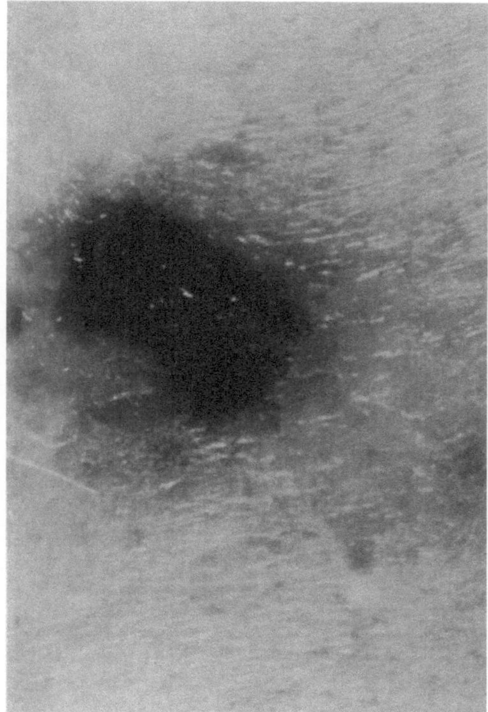

Fig. 34. Basal epithelioma upper back showing diffuse hemorrhagic area after 200 joules exit energy neodymium laser. Area later became atrophic with few areas of telangiectasia

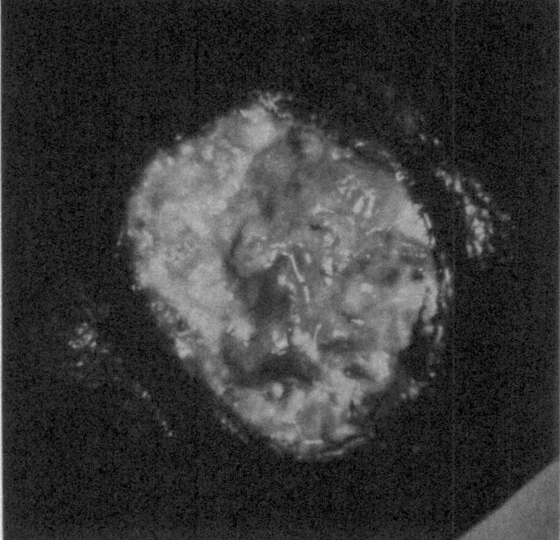

Fig. 35. Recurrent squamous epithelioma of thigh in a Negro after surgery and radiation. Laser impact unfocussed 650 joules exit energy pulsed ruby laser to center and to lower border surface, focussed spot diameter 2 mms, puls duration 3,5 milliseconds and energy density of 20,000 joules/cm². Only effect was immediate softening of the heavy green tenacious slough and dispersion of odorous fragments of slough about the laser laboratory

When investigative studies are completed many of these lesions still may be excised. The first consideration of therapy still should be the therapy which is most suitable for the patient. If laser treatment is given, the initial treatments should be vigorous and adequate as regards energy density of the total lesion.

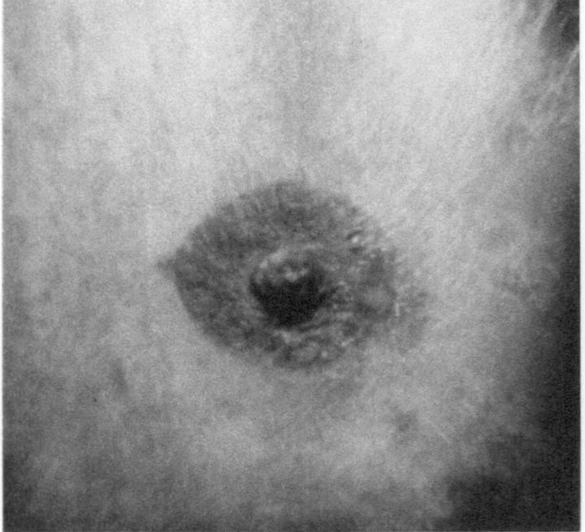

For laser therapy, especially of lesions about the face and neck, protection of the patient should always be considered. The measures usually recommended are of closing the eyes, and then covering all with protective glasses. For impact near the eyes, complete black shutters are used over the glasses.

Protection of the adjacent skin may be secured with such simple measures as cardboard, and drapes — black drapes for the ruby laser and colored drapes for the neodymium laser. In the areas where accurate focusing of impacts is required, the area must be held completely immobile so that there be no movement during impact. As usual, in all forms of laser treatment the protec-

Fig. 36. After impact 300 joules exit energy pulsed ruby laser of cutaneous horn with early squamous carcinoma; area around protected by black paper. Later, entire area desquamated and healed

tion of the operator must also be done with the measures usually recommended. In this field also, it is hoped that laser therapy will be recommended as the therapy of choice for an early lesion in an area where excisional surgery cannot be done or be done only with great difficulty.

Chapter 10

Malignant Lymphomas

Accessible cancer with multiple lesions is a fruitful field for controlled laser cancer research. The malignant lymphoma groups with widespread skin lesions have been used for laser studies. Because of the tendency of spontaneous healing such as even in the tumor phase of mycosis fungoides, control studies must be done.

Laser studies include the effects of different lasers, different energy densities, and focussing at varying depths in the lesions. For example, in a single linear biopsy it is possible to have three areas of different types of impacts — unfocused on surface, focused on surface, and focused 0,5 to 2.0 cms. deep in tissue. These impacts can be placed adjacent to each other and then biopsied so that the microscopic sections contain details in all three areas. HELSPER has done extensive studies with a reticulo-histiocytoma of the skin.

Multiple lesions provide opportunity for investigations with different lasers — ruby, neodymium, and argon gas. These lesions provide also the opportunity for the use of vital dyes. These may be injected locally or even given by perfusions. These dyes are Evan's blue, fluorescein, etc. Indian ink may be injected locally. It is not known whether the laser impact can make dyes cytotoxic or carcinogenic.

The lymphomas provide also an opportunity for experiments on synergism such as Minton, Weiss and Zellen have done with cyclophosphamide and as our laboratory has done with topical nitrogen mustard, topical 5-fluorouracil and 5-desoxyuridine.

The laser may be used also with other topical agents such as dinitrochlorobenzene. Sensitization to dinitrochlorobenzene has been done by van Scott as a therapeutic procedure for mycosis fungoides.

Histological studies of lymphoma show coagulation necrosis of a non-specific type. As yet, studies have not shown any cytologic cellular resistance in the target

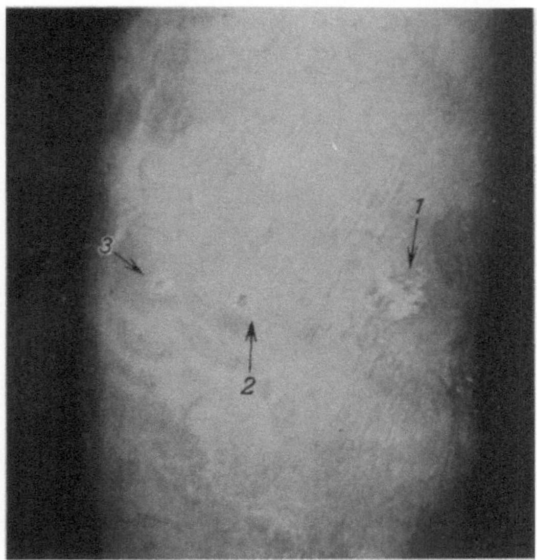

Fig. 37. Placque phase of malignant lymphoma, mycosis fungoides type showing. A. Technique of focussing laser beam through lens. B. 1. unfocussed impact, 2. focussed at surface, 3. focussed 0.5 cm. deep into tissue

area. Healing is localized to the target area only. With superficial reactions, no scarring is produced.

Fresh blood smears of lymphocytic and myelogenous leukemia have been exposed to low energy laser beams, ruby laser, exit energy 3.5 joules, unfocused. Again, the red cells in the field show much worse change than the white cells. However, even these abnormal blood elements do show subtle changes as evident by changes in nuclei after impact.

Experiments have been done also in the exposure of regional lymph glands and the cross firing by the laser beam with focused impacts deep in tissue. These are purely of investigative nature of the study of the local effects of the depth dose.

Some suitable controls in the field of lymphomas include the actual use of xenon light itself and other modalities of radiation given to localized areas. These types of radiation include ultraviolet, thorium x, P^{32}, Sr^{90}, Co^{60} and gamma ray and Grenz ray.

Patients, then with multiple accessible lymphomas offer additional opportunities for controlled studies of laser research on tumors of man. This is much more significant than studies of tumor in animals or in tissue cultures.

Chapter 11

Visceral Malignancies

Experiments with the laser therapy of visceral malignancies have been done mostly with transplanted and spontaneous cancers in animals and with neurosurgery. At the National Cancer Institute, hepatomas in the Rhesus monkey have been treated by high energy neodymium lasers. The hepatomas showed good response and healing with laser treatment. McGuff and Henderson, in our Laboratories, have demon-

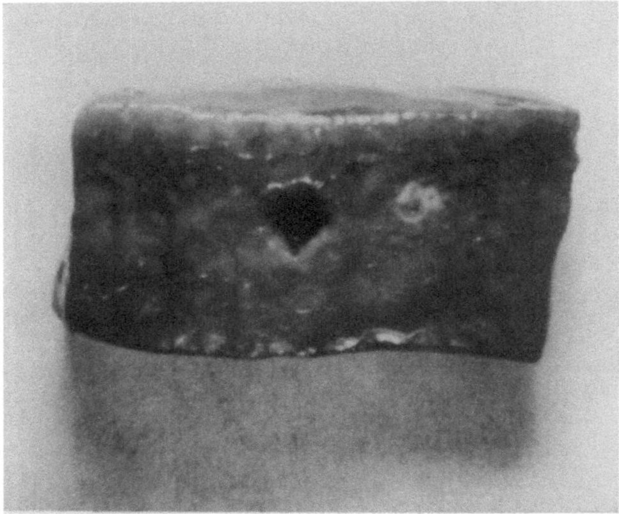

Fig. 38. Human liver tissue showing effect of surface impact ruby laser, superficial charring, and laser transmission deep into liver tissue with quartz glass rod

strated excellent healing of liver impacts in animals after extensive coagulation necrosis by the laser.

Recent developments in the field of high output CW lasers have evoked much interest for laser surgery. Hoye and Minton have used an argon laser for animal surgery. Brown and Henderson of our Laboratory have worked with an argon CW laser with a 2 watt output and also have demonstrated the use, at Bell Laboratories, of the high output argon laser as a precise tool for laser surgery of the skin, subcutaneous tissue, fascia and muscle layers of animals. What is of more interest is the use of the high output argon laser as an optical knife for surgery in such vascular tissues as the liver and lungs. Bleeding is at a minimum with laser surgery with this type of laser. Detailed studies are now under way as regards healing of areas of laser surgery in the liver, spleen, lungs, intestines, etc., and the combined use of adhesive compounds. Eye protection is of considerable concern to the surgeon with the high output CW argon lasers. Light intensity, ultraviolet light, plus high output laser complicate the picture. This requires use of protective screens and heavy multiple protective glasses. Personnel protection, then, must be available so precise surgery can be done with the CW laser. With the increasing development of CW argon lasers to 150 watt outputs, this problem of area and personnel protection is complicated even more. Special fiber optics systems are being used to transmit the argon beam.

The high output CW carbon dioxide and CW nitrogen lasers have not been used as extensively as yet as the argon lasers. In our initial animal studies, high output carbon dioxide laser has an intense thermal effect on tissue. From an economic aspect, the CW lasers are cheaper to produce than high output ruby lasers. For visceral malignancies, then, the CW lasers now appear to be a more precise surgical tool than repetitive neodymium or ruby lasers. Greater flexibility of instrumentation of the CW lasers is needed to take these off the optical bench for the surgeon.

In a patient with an adenocarcinoma of the rectum, McGuff has given laser therapy through a proctoscope and has observed what he considered partial (30%) improvement. The patient later developed extensive spread through the pelvis. Mulvaney in our laboratory is studying the uses of the laser in urologic surgery and in impacts on bladder stones, and in adeno-carcinoma of the bowel metastatic to the vagina and recurrent after radiation.

Because of the relatively low energy treatment requirements in laser neurosurgery, and the opportunities for sharp focussing and the use of quartz rods, delicate laser neurosurgery has been done in dogs. This includes both hypophysectomy and thalamotomy by Brown. Increasing improvement in these quartz rods has made the use of these rods practical in the high energy laser therapy of accessible malignancies of the skin and soft tissues. As Brown indicates, the dog neurosurgery is important for studies of investigations of the effects of the laser. Helmer, in our Laboratory, has done laser impacts on the spinal cord of dogs to attempt to study the possibilities of laser rhizotomy for the relief of the intractable pain of cancer.

The increasing developments of fiber optics to provide fiber optics of sufficient quality to withstand transmission of the laser beam offer a possibility in the operating room of the use of fiber optics for the transmission of laser beams. As yet, this is not possible with fiber optics except for some investigative materials with glass doped with neodymium. Experiments with transmission of argon laser are just beginning. Flexible fiber optics probes may be used in the subcutaneous tissue, the trachea, esophagus, stomach, peritoneal cavity, major bile ducts, middle ear, pelvic cavity, etc. Our Laboratory is developing an operative laser to be used with colpomicroscopy for studies of carcinoma in situ in the cervix. Investigative studies are being done on infrared fiber optics by Kapany for use in remote thermography. This will be of interest in cancer research.

In his initial experiment, Rosomoff used low energy laser systems of 8 joules output for impact of the tumor bed after removal of brain tumors in man. McLaurin and Brown, of our Laboratory, are using high energy laser systems and quartz rods for their investigative studies in laser neurosurgery. The questions of recoil pressure and sonic waves in the brain after laser impact in this area remain to be answered. Barium titanate transducers are used by our Laboratory to monitor impacts about the skull.

4*

As the laser surgical operating room is developed more fully, studies on laser therapy of malignancy will progress. The next field, in order of importance, then, for which laser would be used in man is laser therapy, after laparotomy, for metastatic visceral lesions in the liver, peritoneal cavity and lymph glands. Also, plans have been started for laser treatment of the prostate. Here the need for flexibility of the laser is obvious to be able to reach the mass, to penetrate into the lesion and to avoid damage to adjacent and as yet uninvolved areas such as where major blood vessels or nerves are found.

As plasma torches are developed, these too will be used in the study of visceral malignancies. Plasma torches are gaseous masses of ionized material, electrons and molecules. The temperatures of this mass vary from 40,000 to 60,000° F. The jet velocity of this mass may reach as rapid as 10,000 miles per second. Low temperature

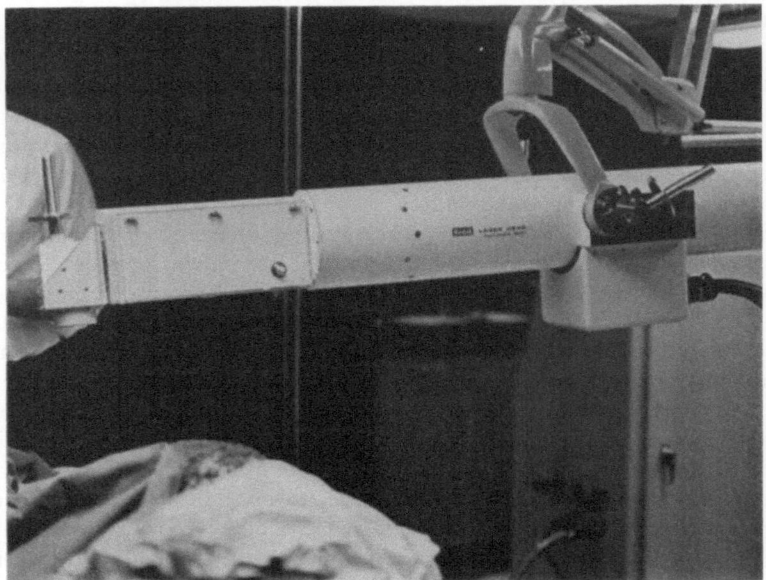

Fig. 39. New experimental Neodymium laser, of Eastman, on treatment stand for increased flexibility for treatment of melanoma. Output 900—1,000 joules exit energy

and low velocity instrumentation are under investigation for biomedical applications. The plasma torch developments are being done by SCHERER and his associates. The plume of the laser is a type of plasma and has some superficial relationship to the plasma of the plasma torch. The plasma torch will be used as one of the control techniques for laser surgery. As indicated previously, our initial studies with the plasma torch are as controls for the high output carbon dioxide laser.

The initial studies of visceral laser surgery, then, will be done on the metastatic lesions of widespread visceral malignancies. Then hopefully will follow adequate and effective laser therapy for the early lesion. If the surgical operation of the early lesion cannot be done adequately with excision or electrosurgery, then laser surgery can be done. At present, if high energy laser systems are used, the entire lesions should be covered with impacts, when this can be done. If focused as well as unfocused beams are to be used, the focused impacts should be done first so that maximum energy density is available for depth as well as for the surface.

The future of laser therapy of visceral malignancies will be related to progress and developments of the laser operating room. Problems of laser surgery in the operating room in regard to what is called so often and discouragingly, "the present state of the art", are many. The instrument must have a high output, be flexible and easily controlled by the surgeon, maintain sterility precautions and be safe for operation as regards electrical and anesthesia hazards.

At present, our laser operating rooms have 650 joules exit energy ruby lasers, a laboratory model of an 1160 exit energy neodymium laser on loan from the Eastman Kodak Company and a 2—10 watt CW argon laser on loan from the Bell Telephone Laboratories. The ruby laser is flexible, not as yet under the direct control of the surgeon but able to be moved in all planes by the technician. The neodymium laser loaned by Eastman is flexible but the argon lasers are less flexible. However, our Laboratory, in conjunction with Applied Lasers, Inc., is developing a flexible, moveable laser treatment stand for the operating room. Power supply units are kept out of the operating room.

At the National Cancer Institute in Washington, D. C., under the direction of KETCHAM, is a high energy flexible neodymium laser, 800 joules exit energy, in a specially constructed laser surgical operating room. This is under the direct control of the operating surgeon. This has just begun to be used. The total cost of this laser surgical area is much in excess of $ 500,000.00.

Halothane anesthesia may be used in general surgery with lasers. In general, any anesthesia which may be used for electro-surgery can be used for laser surgery. With special drapes and an experienced operating room team, sterility can be maintained.

Personnel protection also must be maintained through training, monitoring of the instrumentation, and the continued use of uncomfortable protective glasses.

Chapter 12

Investigative Studies on the Possible Carcinogenic Action of the Laser

One of the hazards to be considered in laser therapy is the possibility of the carcinogenic property of the laser itself. Since this is a form of radiation, although mostly visible light, studies in carcinogenic properties should be considered. As yet, there is no evidence, that laser radiation is carcinogenic, even in animals used in laser experiments.

Our clinical observations are based on over 200 patients who have been treated in the past four years with laser for many benign conditions as part of investigative studies. Such studies have been on patients with normal skin, patients with benign skin diseases for which some forms of radiation are usually helpful, such as warts, chronic intractable neurodermatitis and psoriasis.

In one laser investigator, an atopic with reactive skin, low energy laser impacts in the range of 50 joules/cm² of pulsed ruby laser have been given almost daily repeatedly for the past four years to normal skin of the flexor surface of the forearm. Early in the course of the study one impact of high energy laser said to be 90 joules exit energy produced four days after impact some bizarre mitoses in the epidermis as well as thrombosis of the superficial vessels of the dermis. Repeated impacts of the laser in this individual with energy densities as high as 1,000 to 2,000 joules/cm² with the pulsed ruby laser did not produce evidence of malignant change with the impact area observed for several years. Recently his minimal reactive dose with the pulsed ruby laser has been reduced to 38 joules/cm² 0.05 mm² target area pulse duration 1 millisecond. Attempts to induce this increased reactivity in other individuals receiving repeated laser impacts were not successful. However, as yet, no patients with atopy have been studied.

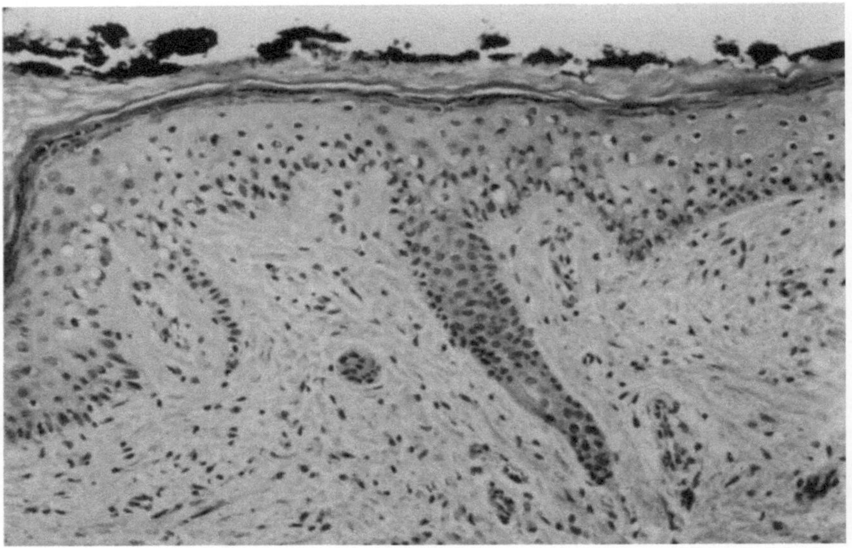

Fig. 40. Follow-up biopsy of nodular basal cell epithelioma right wrist 110 days after laser treatment showing absence of tumor and non-specific fibrosis and basophilic degeneration of collagen. Color on top is silver sulphide tatoo to orient thin biopsy fragment. Hematoxylin-eosin × 90. (From S.A.M.A. 189; 714, 1964 treatment of basal cell epithelioma by laser radiation. L. GOLDMAN and R. G. WILSON)

Investigative studies were done with removal of tattoo marks in two patients. These individuals have been subjected repeatedly to laser radiation over a period of several years. Energy densities varied in these patients from 75 joules/exit energy to 250 joules/exit energy from ruby laser and 370 joules/exit energy from neodymium. First, hypertrophic scarring then smooth scarring resulted. The scars have been observed for more than a year. Biopsies, to date, have shown non-specific fibrosis with retained fragments of the tattoo material and no evidence of malignant degeneration. In treatment of psoriasis and warts by the laser no abnormal changes were noticed in the skin after low energy impacts. The patients in this series have been observed for a period of only two years. Recently, a large series of patients has been treated for the removal of their tattoo marks with ruby, neodymium and argon lasers. Cancer does occur in burn scars. Most of these according to GIBLIN, PICKRELL, PITTS, and ARMSTRONG require twenty to thirty years or more after the burn to develop. Scars in post radiation areas may develop earlier.

Impacts of normal skin with the high energy laser using Q-switching techniques, 85 megawatts peak power outputs, have been studied for electron spin resonance spectrometry. To-date, the studies on our series have been done by Jocobi and have shown no evidence of free radicle formation has been detected by Derr, Klein and Fine in black skin of animals but not in white skin. It is obvious that these clinical progress reports are preliminary in nature and have not been followed up for long periods of time. It is emphasized that these studies in our laboratory were done on skin of individuals not on excised material.

To attempt to induce cancer in animals, McGuff and Ritter of our Laboratory have exposed animals — white rats, guinea pigs and hamsters — to single high energy impacts more than 50 joules/exit energy and to repeated exposures to low energy 1 to 3 joules/exit energy ruby and neodymium lasers. Studies will be done

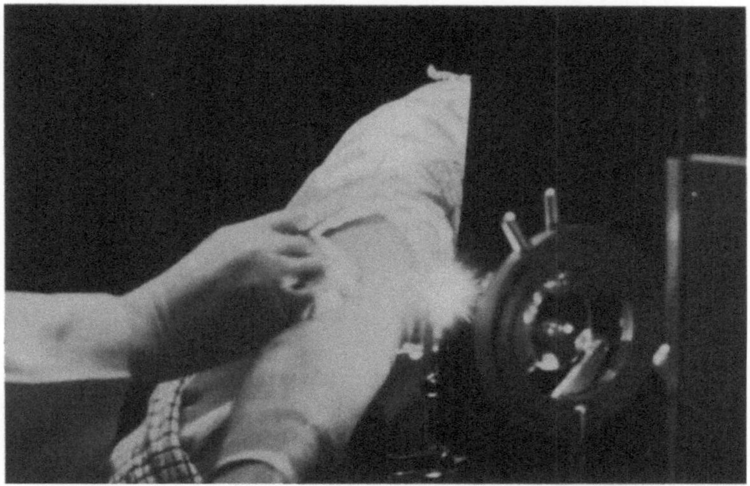

Fig. 41. Q-switched ruby laser 85 megawatts peak power output cooled immediately with wave nitrogen excised for ESR studies which were negative

also on single and repeated impacts on skin colored by various dyes. As yet, their studies show no positive findings in unselected strains. Studies with laser impact on hairless mice, a more fruitful source of tumors induced by radiation, have been initiated recently.

Studies of the laser as a cocarcinogen with painting with methyl-cholanthrene, exposure to x-ray, Grenz, xenon, and ultra violet light, have also been started recently. These studies are done because of the combined uses of laser therapy with other modalities of radiation and with local and systemic cancer chemotherapy.

Tissue culture techniques by Rounds and his associates and by Malt may also reveal potential carcinogenic features of laser impacts. Detailed controls are needed. Only rarely have chromosomal aberrations been observed in tissue cultures following laser impacts. All this incomplete data means that follow-up studies are needed both in experimental animals and in man. Clinical investigative studies on man must continue as indicated repeatedly. The limitation of the use of the laser to conditions for which laser therapy is indicated for investigative purposes will avoid indiscriminate careless use. Of necessity, the limitation of at least the high energy laser studies to large medical centers will assure some measure of critical control of this important investigative surgical instrument.

Chapter 13

Future Needs for Clinical Investigative Studies

It is obvious from this brief survey of laser cancer research that many studies are partially or wholly incomplete probing often of a superficial pilot type of experiments. These attempt to indicate only trends of investigative studies. To forestall the cries of the disturbed and wholly justified critics, it is admitted that, at present per-

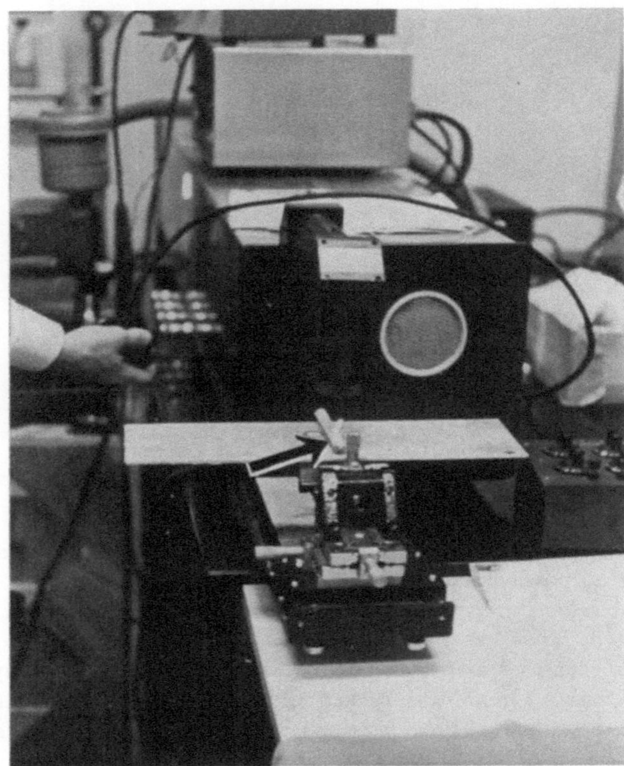

Fig. 42. Experimental model, continuous wave (CW) carbon dioxide laser, 106,000 Å, from Perkin-Elmer-Corporation. 10 Watt output on section of fibula, showing impact with flame at site of impact. Beam is invisible

haps, not even a monograph on the laser is warranted. However, the laser is here. It is more than ready and willing to move out of the physics laboratory and from the area of applied physical science. Also, many studies have been done already. Many of these are basic and well controlled. It is now time to study man.

The research worker in cancer must evaluate the laser in all its phases. In the laboratory, the laser attached to the microscope is used for studies in cancer cytology and cytogenetics. In the chemistry laboratory, the laser is used to study dyes, photochemical reactions and spectroscopy (even of living cancer tissue!). In the experimental animal with acquired or transplanted cancer, laser surgery is added to other experimental surgical techniques. In the cancer treatment center, the laser is here now ready to be used as another type of surgery. The oncologist has always had to learn many other disciplines and had to supervise many other disciplines of medicine. Now, he has the laser.

It is emphasized that this optical knife is a surgical tool not just another gadget for the radiobiologist. Now, it is the surgeon who must learn this radiation therapy and to make lesions accessible to its incident beam. Now in the operating room with him are physicists and engineers to monitor, even operate and modify this tool.

To give him continued skill and assurance in the operating room with the laser, many things will have to be done and many studies will have to be continued. In brief, these are in summary:

1. continued interest of the manufacturer to develop reliable safe instrumentation with ruby and neodymium lasers with constant range of output especially for high energy and high peak power levels for actual operating room use;
2. to continue research in high output gas lasers as the argon, carbon dioxide and ultraviolet lasers and to learn eye protection for the operating surgeon;
3. to continue research on reliable and reproducible techniques of measurement of laser output so that standardized dosage data maybe exchanged between laser treatment centers;
4. to continue basic studies on the mechanism of the laser reaction at cellular level in living tissue of man and animals. These basic studies should include biochemical, biophysical and immunobiologic investigations;
5. to continue studies on the use of pigments for the cancer and even for the regional lymph nodes to increase absorption of the laser beam;
6. to continue studies on the mechanism of the laser reaction in cancer tissue as regards hyperthermia, pressure and ultra-sonic waves, charged particles, etc.;
7. to continue controlled studies on the surgical uses of the laser in primary and metastatic cancer with controls of the knife, electrosurgery used where possible, plasma torch and cryosurgery;
8. to continue studies of the use of the laser as an adjunct for cancer radiation with other modalities of radiation and for cancer chemotherapy, both local and systemic;
9. to provide for long term studies of the laser treated patient as regards the treatment of the local area and his systemic reactions;
10. to continue studies on area and personal protection of patient and laser personnel;
11. to have international committees of laser research and laser treatments to collect, analyze and evaluate data and to make recommendations;
12. to encourage physicists to continue basic research in laser physics and to make them aware of the interest and significance of biomedical applications.

So, here is another challenge for cancer therapy. This tool, is still immature but is expensive, sophisticated, and mostly untried but already shows some encouraging results in the therapy of accessible cancer in man. The future depends on much co-operative and basic, clinical research by dedicated and critical investigators who have the fortunate opportunity to work with the laser as it develops.

References

AMY, ROBERT L, and R. STORB: Selective mitochondrial damage by a ruby laser microbeam: An electron microscopic study. Science 150, 756 (1965).

BAEZ, S., and J. P. KOCHEN: Laser induced microagglutination in an isolated vascular model system. Ann. N. Y. Acad. Sci. 122, 738 (1965).

BARNES, F., J. DANIEL, and K. TAKAHASHI: Laser surgery and biological damage. Presented at NEREM, Boston, November (1965).

BASOV, N. G.: Semiconductor lasers. Science 149, 821 (1965).

— and A. M. PROKHOROV: Applications of molecular beams to radio spectroscopic studies of rotation spectra of molecules. Physics USSR 101, 47 (1955a).

BENNETT, W. R., jr.: Excitation and inversion mechanisms in gas lasers. Ann. N. Y. Acad. Sci. 122, 579 (1965).

BERKOWITZ, J., and W. A. CHUPKA: Mass spectrometric study of vapor ejected from graphite and other solids by focused laser beams. J. Chem. Phys. 40, 2735 (1964).

BESSIS, M., F. GIRES, G. MAYER, and G. NOMARSKI: Irradiation des organites cellulaires à l'aide d'un laser à rubis. C. R. Acad. Sci. (Paris). 255, 1010 (1962).

— and M. TER-POGOSSIAN: Micropuncture of cells by means of a laser beam. Ann. N. Y. Acad. Sci. 122, 659 (1965).

BRECH, F., and L. CROSS: Optical microemission stimulated by a ruby maser. Appl. Spectrosc. 16, 59 (1962).

BURKHALTER, J. H.: Material effects of laser radiation and basic interaction phenomena. Fed. Proc. 24, 31 (1965).

CAMPBELL, C. J., K. S. NOYORI, M. C. RITTLER, and C. J. KOESTER: Clinical use of the laser retinal photocoagulator. Fed. Proc. 24, 71 (1965).

— — — — Retinal coagulation: Clinical studies. Ann. N. Y. Acad. Sci. 122, 780 (1965).

—, M. C. RITTLER, and C. J. KOESTER: The optical maser as a retinal coagulator: An evaluation. Trans. Amer. Acad. Ophthalmol. Otolaryngol. 67, 58 (1963).

CULLOM, J. H., and R. W. WAYNANT: Determination of laser damage threshold for various glasses. Appl. Opt. 3, 989 (1964).

DERR, V. E., E. KLEIN, and S. FINE: Free radical occurrence in some laser irradiated biologic materials. Fed. Proc. 24, 99 (1965).

EARLE, K. M., D. STERLING, U. ROSSMAN, M. A. ROSS, J. R. HAYNES, and E. H. ZEITLER: Central nervous system effects of laser radiation. Fed. Proc. 24, 129 (1965).

EINSTEIN, A.: Zur Quantentheorie der Strahlung. Phys. Zeit. 18, 121 (1917).

FERGUSON, H. S., J. E. MENTALL, and R. W. NICHOLLS: Laser excitation of powdered solids. Nature 204, 1295 (1964).

FINE, S., and E. KLEIN: Biological effects of laser radiation, management study submitted to U. S. Air Force Missile Development Center, Air Force Systems Command, United States Air Force, Washington, D. S. (1965).

— —, and Y. LAOR: Modification of effects of laser radiation by light absorbing chemicals, presented at Boston Laser Conf. 3rd, Boston, Massachusetts, August 5 (1964).

—, W. NOWAK, W. HANSEN, K. KERGENROTHER, R. E. SCOTT, J. DONOGHUE, and E. DERR: Interaction of laser radiation with biologic systems, I. Studies on interaction with tissues. Fed. Proc. 24, 25 (1965).

— —, and R. E. SCOTT: Laser irradiation of biological systems. IEEE Spectrum 1, 81 (April 1964).

— — —, Y. LAOR, L. SIMPSON, J. CRISSEY, J. DONOGHUE, and V. E. KLEIN: Measurements and hazards on interaction of laser radiation and biological systems. NEREM Record 6, 158 (1964).

FREEMAN, H. M., O. POMERANTZEFF, and C. SCHEPENS: Retinal laser coagulations: clinical studies, N. Y. Acad. Sci. 122, 783 (1965).

GEERAETS, W. J., W. T. HAM, jr., R. C. WILLIAMS, H. A. MUELLER, J. BURKHART, D. GUEERY III, and J. J. VOS: Laser versus light coagulator: A funduscopic and histologic study of chorioretinal injury as a function of exposure time. Fed. Proc. 24, 48 (1965).

—, R. C. WILLIAMS, G. CHAN, W. T. HAM, jr., D. GUEERY, III, and E. H. SCHMIDT: The loss of light energy in retina and choroid. Arch. Ophthalmol. 64, 606 (1960).

GIBLIN, T., K. PICKRELL, W. PITTS, and D. ARMSTRONG: Malignant degeneration in burn scars: Marjohn's ulcer. Ann. Surg. 162, 291 (1965).

GOLDMAN, J., P. HORNBY, and C. LONG: Effect of the laser beam on the skin: Transmission of laser beams through fiber optics. J. invest. Derm. 42, 231 (1964).

—, and R. MEYER: Transmission of laser beams through various transparent rods for biomedical applications. Nature 205, 4974; 892 (1964).

GOLDMAN, L.: Comparison of the biomedical effects of the exposure of human tissues to low and high energy lasers. Ann. N. Y. Acad. Sci. 122, 802 (1965).

— Dermatologic manifestations of laser radiation. Fed. Proc. 24, 1 (1965).

— Derzeitige Untersuchungen von dermatologischem Interesse mit dem Laser. Hautarzt (1965).

— Experiences with treatment of patients with high energy ruby and neodymium lasers. Presented at NEREM, November (1965).

— Protection of personnel operating lasers. American Journal of Medical Electronics 2, 335 (1963).

— The laser in medical research and surgery. The New Scientist 21, 284 (1964).

—, D. J. BLANEY, A. FREEMOND, and P. HORNBY: The biomedical aspects of lasers. J. Amer. med. Assoc. 188, 302 (1964).

— —, D. J. KINDEL III., E. K. FRANKE, and ING.: Effect of laser beam on the skin: Preliminary report. J. invest. Derm. 40, 121 (1963).

— — —, D. RICHFIELD, E. FRANKE: Pathology of the effect of the laser beam on the skin. Nature 19, 912 (1963).

— — — —, P. OWENS, and E. HOMANS: Effect of the laser beam on the skin: Exposure of cytological preparations. J. invest. Derm. 42, 247 (1964).

—, T. BROWN, P. HORNBY, J. ROCKWELL, and R. MEYER: Investigative studies with quartz rods for high energy laser transmission. Amer. J. med. Electronics, in press.

—, J. A. GRAY, B. GOLDMAN, and R. MEYER: Effect of laser beam impacts on teeth. J. Amer. dent. Assoc. 70, 601 (1965).

—, G. A. HARDWAY, and B. KRASHES: Preliminary studies on the use of the laser in lapidary work. Lapidary Journ. (1963).

—, and P. HORNBY: The design of a medical laser laboratory. Arch. environm. Hth 10, 493 (1965).

— —, R. MEYER, and B. GOLDMAN: Impact of the laser on dental caries. Nature 203, 417 (1964).

—, J. IGELMAN, and D. RICHFIELD: Impact of the laser on nevi and melanomas. Arch. Derm. 90, 71 (1964).

—, and P. OWENS: Chromosome studies in dermatology; Preliminary observations in some congenital and acquired dermatoses and in the effect of radiations with x-ray, grenz ray, and laser. Acta derm.-venereol. (Stockh.) 44, 268 (1964).

—, and D. RICHFIELD: The effect of repeated exposures to laser beams. Acta derm.-venereol. (Stockh.) 44, 264 (1964).

—, and R. WILSON: Treatment of basal cell epithelioma by laser radiation. J. Amer. med. Assoc. 188, 773 (1964).

— —, P. HORNBY, and R. MEYER: Radiation from a Q-switched laser with a total power output of 10 megawatts on a tattoo of man. J. invest. Derm. 44, 69 (1965).

— — — — Laser radiation of malignancy in man. Cancer 18, 533 (1965).

— — — — The biomedical aspects of laser. Exhibit presented at AMA Annual Convention June (1965).

HAM, W. T.: Ocular radiation effects. Boston Laser Conference 2nd Northeastern University, Boston, Mass. (1963).

HANSEN, W. P., S. FINE, G. R. PEACOCK, and E. KLEIN: Focusing of laser light by target surfaces and effects on initial temperature conditions. Presented at NEREM, November, Boston (1965).

HARDWAY, G.: Q-switching. Ann. N. Y. Acad. Sci. 122, 608 (1965).

HARPER, D. W.: Laser damage in glasses. Brit. J. appl. Phys. 16, 751 (1965).

HEAVENS, O. S.: Optical masers. London: Methuen and Co., Ltd. 1964.

HELSPER, J. T., G. S. SHARP, H. F. WILLIAMS, and H. W. FISTER: The biological effect of laser energy on human melanoma. Cancer 17, 1299—1304 (Nov. 1964).

HELWIG, E., W. JONES, J. HAYES, and E. ZEITLER: Anatomic and histochemical changes in skin after laser irradiation. Fed. Proc. 24, 583 (1965).

IGELMAN, J. M., and T. ROTTE: Effects of laser radiation on tyrosinase. Fed. Proc. 24, 94 (1965).

— —, E. SCHECHTER, and D. J. BLANEY: Exposure of enzymes to laser radiation. Ann. N. Y. Acad. Sci. 122, 790 (1965).

JAVAN, A., W. R. BENNET, jr., and D. R. HERRIOTT: Population inversion and continuous optical maser oscillation in gas discharge containing a HeNE mixture. Phys. Rev. 6, 106 (1961).

KANTOR, Z., I. KAPLAN, E. GRUENBERG, and S. GITTER: Antigenic properties of burnt skin. Nature 207, 540 (1965).

KETCHAM, A., and J. MINTON: Laser radiation as a clinical tool in cancer therapy. Fed. Proc. 24, 159 (1965).

KLEIN, E., Y. C. LOAR, L. C. SIMPSON, S. FINE, J. EDLOW, and M. LITWIN: Threshold studies and reversible depigmentation in rodent skin. Presented at NEREM, Boston, Mass. November (1965).

KOCHEN, J. A., and S. BAEZ: Laser induced micro vascular thrombosis embolization and recanalization in the rat. Ann. N. Y. Acad. Sci. 122, 728 (1965).

KOESTER, C. J., E. SNITZER, C. J. CAMPBELL, and M. C. RITTLER: Experimental laser retina coagulator. J. Opt. Soc. Am. 52, 607 (1962).

—, M. R. THORBURN, H. JUPNIK, and C. J. CAMPBELL: Design and performance of a laser photocoagulator. Presented at NEREM, Boston, Mass. November (1965).

Laser Data Compilation, Maser Optics, Maser Optics, Inc.

LAX, B.: Semiconductor lasers. Ann. N. Y. Acad. Sci. 122, 598 (1965).

LINLOR, W. J.: Ion energies produced by laser giant pulse. Appl. Phys. Let. 3, 310 (1963).

LITHWICK, N., M. HEALY, and J. COHEN: Microanalysis of bone by laser microprobe. Surg. Form 15, 439 (1964).

LITWIN, M., and D. GLEW: Biological effects of laser radiation. J. Amer. med. Soc. 187, 842 (1964).

MAIMAN, T. H.: Stimulated optical radiation in ruby masers. Nature 187, 493 (1960).

MALT, R.: Effects of laser radiation on subcellular components. Fed. Proc. 24, 122 (1965).

—, and C. H. TOWNES: Optical masers in biology and medicine. New Engl. J. Med. 269, 1417 (1963).

McGUFF, P.: Effects of laser radiation on tumor transplants. Fed. Proc. 24, 150 (1965).

— Bio-engineering aspects of laser radiation. Presented at NEREM, Boston, Mass. Nov. (1965).

— Surgical applications of the laser (in press).

—, D. BUSHNELL, H. SOROFF, and R. DETERLING, jr.: Studies of surgical applications of laser. Surg. For. 14, 143 (1963).

— R. A. DETERLING, jr., L. S. GOTTLIEB, H. D. FAHIMI, D. BUSHNELL, and F. ROEBER: The laser treatment of experimental malignant tumors. Canadian Medical Association Journal 91, 1089—1095 November (1964).

— — —, D. BUSNELL, and F. ROEBER: Laser radiation of malignancies. Ann. N. Y. Acad. Sci. 122, 747 (1965).

MENDELSON, J. A., and N. B. ACKERMAN: Studies of biologically significant forces following laser irradiation. Fed. Proc. 24, 111 (1965).

MENTALL, J. E., and R. W. NICHOLLS: Temperature measurements on laser-produced flames. Presented at Spring Meeting, Am. Phys. Soc. Washington, D. C. April (1965).

MINTON, J. P.: Some factors affecting tumor response after laser radiation. Fed. Proc. 24, 155 (1965).

—, and M. ZELEN: Oncolysis with laser energy combined with chemotherapy. Nature 207, 140 (1965).

— —, and A. S. KETCHAM: Experimental results from exposure of Cloudman S-91 melanoma in the CDBA/2F$_1$ hybrid mouse to neodymium or ruby laser radiation. Ann. N. Y. Acad. Sci. 122, 758 (1965).

NOWAK, W. B., S. FINE, E. KLEIN, K. HERGENROTHER, and W. P. HANSEN: On the use of thermocouples for temperature measurement during laser irradiation. Life Science 3, 1475 (1964).

PAO, Y. H., and P. M. RENTZEPIS: Laser-induced production of free radicals in organic compounds. Appl. Phys. Let. 6, 93 (1965).

READY, J. F.: Effects due to absorption of laser radiation. J. appl. Phys. 36, 462 (1965).

RENTZEPIS, P. M., and Y. H. PAO: Multiphoton processes in photochemistry. Abst. 149th Meeting Am. Chem. Soc. Abst. 4, 21 (1965).

ROSAN, R., F. BRECH, and D. GLICK: Current problems in laser microprobe analysis. Fed. Proc. 24, 126 (1965).

—, M. HEALY, and W. McNARY: Spectroscopic ultramicroanalysis with a laser. Science 143, 236 (1963).

ROSAN, R. C.: On the preparation of samples for laser microprobe analysis. Appl. Spectrosc. 19, 97 (1965).

ROUNDS, D. E.: Effects of laser radiation on cellcultures. Fed. Proc. 24, 116 (1965).

—, and J. E. ADAMS: DNA metabolism in synchronized mamalian cells following laser radiation. Boston Laser Conf. 3rd, Northeastern University, Boston, Mass. (1964).

—, J. BOOKER, F. F. STRASSER, and R. S. OLSON: The potentiation of gamma radiation with energy from a ruby laser. Technical Documentary Report No. SAM-TDR No. 115 102.

—, and E. C. CHAMBERLAIN: Preliminary observations of the effects of laser irradiation on cells grown in tissue cultures. Boston Laser Conf. 2nd, Northeastern University, Boston, Mass. (1963).

— —, and T. OKIGAKI: Laser radiation of tissue cultures. Ann. N. Y. Acad. Sci. 122, 713 (1964).

—, R. S. OLSON, and F. M. JOHNSON: The effect of the laser on cellular respiration. Presented at NEREM, Boston, Mass., November (1965).

RUNGE, E. F., R. W. MINCK, and F. R. BRYAN: Spectrochemical analysis using a pulsed laser source. Spectrochem. ACTA. 20, 733 (1964).

SAKS, N., C. ROTH, and A. CHARLES: Ruby laser as amicrosurgical instrument. Science 141, 46 (1963).

SAKS, N. M., R. C. ZUZOLO, and M. J. KOPAC: Microsurgery of living cells by ruby laser erracication. N. Y. Acad. Sci. 122, 695 (1965).

SCHEPENS, and H. FREEMAN: Studies on laser photocoagulation. Presented at Conf. Biol. Effects Laser Radiation. Med. Phys. Soc. Boston, Mass. (1963).

SCHNIEPER, P. A.: Flash photolysis — An application of electrical engineering in chemical research. Presented at NEREM, Boston, Mass. November (1965).

SHAWLOW, A. L., and C. H. TOWNES: Infrared and optical masers. C. H. Phys. Rev. 112, 1940 (1958).

SHERMAN, D. B., M. P. RUBEN, and H. M. GOLDMAN: The application of laser for the spectrochemical analysis of calcified tissues. Ann. N. Y. Acad. Sci. 122, 767 (1965).

SOLON, L. R., R. AARONSON, and G. GOULD: Physiological implications of laser beams. Science 134, 1506 (1961).

STRATTON, K., M. A. PATHAK, and S. FINE: ESR studies of melanin containing tissues after laser irradiation. Presented at NEREM, Boston, Mass. November (1965).

STRAUB, H. W.: Protection of the human eye from laser radiation, TR-1153 Harry Diamond Laboratories, Army Material Commands, Washington, D. C., July (1963).

— Protection of the human eye from laser radiation. Ann. N. Y. Acad. Sci. 122, 773 (1965).

SUCSY, L. G.: Masers and Lasers, Cambridge, Mass. Maser/Laser Associates (1962).

TOMBERG, V.: Non-thermal effects of laser beams. Nature 204, 868 (1964).

TOWNES, C. H.: Optical masers and their possible application in biology. Biophys. J. 2, 325 (1962).
— Optical and infrared maser. M.I.T. Symposium (1964).
VALI, W.: On the production of high energy particles by giant pulse lasers. IEEE Proc. May (1965).
WEBER, J.: Amplification of microwave radiation by substances not in thermal Equilibrium. Trans. Instit. Radio Engr. Professional Group on Electronic Services. 3, 1 (1953).
— Masers. Rev. Mod. Phys. 31, 681 (1959).
— Some notes on lasers: Concluding remarks. Ann. N. Y. Acad. Sci. 22, 571 (1965).
WILEY, R. H.: Laser organic chemistry. Ann. N. Y. Acad. Sci. 122, 685 (1965).
ZARET, M. M.: Analysis of factors of laser radiation producing retinal damage. Fed. Proc. 24, 62 (1965).
—, G. M. BREININ, H. SCHMIDT, H. RIPPS, I. SIEGEL, and L. R. SOLON: Ocular lesions produced by an optical maser (laser). Science 134, 525 (1961).
—, H. RIPPS, I. M. SIEGEL, and G. BREININ: Laser photocoagulation of the eye. Arch. Ophthalmol. 69, 97 (1963).

Monographs already published

SCHINDLER, R., Lausanne: Die tierische Zelle in Zellkultur (Volume 1).

Neuroblastomas — Biochemical Studies. Edited by C. BOHUON, Villejuif (Volume 2, Symposium).

HUEPER, W. C., Bethesda: Occupational and Environmental Cancers of the Respiratory System (Volume 3).

GOLDMAN, L., Cincinnati: Laser Cancer Research (Volume 4).

Malignant Transformation by Viruses. Edited by W. H. KIRSTEN, Chicago (Volume 6, Symposium).

In production

METCALF, D., Melbourne: The Thymus. Its Role in Immune Responses, Leukemia Development and Carcinogenesis (Volume 5).

MOERTEL, CH. G., Rochester: Multiple Primary Malignant Neoplasms: Their Incidence and Significance (Volume 7).

New Trends in the Treatment of Cancer. Edited by L. MANUILA, S. MOLES and P. RENTCHNICK, Genève (Volume 8, Symposium).

LINDENMANN, J., Zürich / A. KLEIN, Gainesville, Florida: Immunity to Transplantable Tumors following Viral Oncolysis (Volume 9).

NELSON, R. S., Houston: Radioactive Phosphorus in the Diagnosis of Gastrointestinal Cancer (Volume 10).

FREEMANN, R. G., Houston/J. M. KNOX, Paris: Treatment of Skin Cancer (Volume 11).

In preparation

DENOIX, P., Villejuif: Le traitement des cancers du sein.

FISHER, E. R., Pittsburgh: Ultrastructure of Human Normal and Neoplastic Prostate.

FUCHS, W. A., Bern: Lymphography and Tumordiagnosis.

GRUNDMANN, E., Wuppertal-Elberfeld: Morphologie und Cytochemie der Carcinogenese.

HALPERN, B., Paris / PEJSACHOWICZ, Paris: L'agrégation des cellules cancéreuses in vitro.

HAYWARD, J. L., London: Cancer of the Breast: Hormonal Changes.

KERN, G., Köln: Carcinoma in situ.

MARTZ, G., Zürich: Hormonbehandlung der Tumoren.

MATHÉ, G., Villejuif: Les essais d'éradication des leucémies aiguës.

NEWMAN, M. K., Detroit: Neuropathies and Myopathies associated with Occult Malignancies.

PACK, G. T., New York: Clinical Aspects of Cancer Immunity and Cancer Suscepti-
bility.
PACK, G. T., New York / A. H. ISLAMI, New York: Tumors of the Liver.
RITZMAN, S. E., Galveston / W. C. LEVIN, Galveston: The Syndrome of Macroglobuli-
nemia.
STEWARD, J. K., Manchester: Tumors in Children.
WEIL, R., Lausanne: Biological and structural properties of polyoma virus and its
DNA.
ZILBER, L. A., Moskva: Virogenetic Theory of Cancer Origin.

Herstellung: Konrad Triltsch, Graphischer Betrieb, Würzburg